Selected Proceedings of the Fifth Baveno International Consensus Workshop

FIFTH EDITION

EDITED BY

Roberto de Franchis, MD, AGAF

Department of Medical Sciences, University of Milan, and
Gastroenterology 3 Unit, IRCCS Ca' Granda Ospedale Maggiore Policlinico
Mangiagalli and Regina Elena Foundation, Milan, Italy

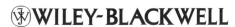

A John Wiley & Sons, Ltd., Publication

Reprinted from

Portal Hypertension V: Proceedings of the Fifth Baveno International Consensus Workshop

ISBN: 9781444334494

© 2011 Blackwell Publishing Ltd

Printed and bound in Great Britain by TJ International Ltd, Padstow, Cornwall

Contents

Preface

Portal hypertension is associated with the most severe complications of cirrhosis, including ascites, hepatic encephalopathy and bleeding from gastro-oesophageal varices. Despite the progress achieved over the last decades, the six-week mortality associated with variceal bleeding is still in the order of 10–20%. Awareness of the difficulty inherent to the evaluation of diagnostic tools and the design and conduct of good clinical trials for the treatment of portal hypertension has led to the organization of a series of consensus meetings. The first one was organized in 1986 in Groningen, The Netherlands by Andrew Burroughs. After Groningen, other meetings followed, in Baveno in 1990 (Baveno I) and 1995 (Baveno II), in Milan in 1992, in Reston, USA, in 1996, in Stresa in 2000 (Baveno III), again in Baveno in 2005 (Baveno IV), and in Atlanta, USA in 2007.

The aims of these meetings were to develop definitions of key events in portal hypertension and variceal bleeding, to review the existing evidence on the natural history, the diagnosis and the therapeutic modalities of portal hypertension and to issue evidence-based recommendations for the conduct of clinical trials and the management of patients. All these meetings were successful and produced consensus statements on some important points, although some issues remained unsettled.

To continue the work of the previous meetings, with the help and encouragement of a group of friends from 14 countries, many of whom had taken part in the previous four Baveno meetings, we organized a Baveno V workshop which took place in Stresa on May 21–22, 2010.

The aims of the Baveno V workshop were the same as in Baveno I–IV, namely, to refine and extend the definitions of key events concerning the bleeding episode, in the light of the feedback we had received from studies carried out after Baveno IV, and to reassess the diagnostic tools and the therapeutic options in patients with portal hypertension. In addition, we continued the effort that was begun in Groningen and continued in the following workshops, of producing updated guidelines aimed at improving the quality of our future studies and of patients' care in general. We were very fortunate in being able to bring to these workshops many of the experts responsible for most of the major achievements of the last years in this field.

The structure of the Baveno V workshop included two symposia, five consensus sessions, eight lectures and a report from paediatrics. The symposia were devoted to the evaluation of the new diagnostic tools that have been developed or refined in the last few years and of the new treatment options that have appeared on the horizon. Of the five sessions, one concerned the definition of key events of the bleeding episode, three covered the therapeutic options in patients with portal hypertension, and the fifth was dedicated to non-cirrhotic portal hypertension. The eight lectures were different in scope: the first one was introductory and summarized the past history of the Baveno workshops and the impact that the publications derived from these workshops have had on the medical literature. In addition, it outlined what needs to be done in the future if the Baveno tradition is to continue. The second lecture was of a methodological nature and described the types and uses of endpoints in clinical trials. The third, fourth, fifth, sixth and seventh lectures addressed important clinical issues, such as the opportunity to use prognostic variables to direct therapy of the acute bleeding episode, the state of advancement in the validation of the stages classification of cirrhosis, the coagulopathy of cirrhosis, the use of anticoagulant therapy in cirrhosis with portal vein thrombosis, and the relationship between variceal bleeding, infection and the hepatorenal stndrome. The eighth lecture outlines the differences and similarities between adult and paediatric portal hypertension, and reported a survey of paediatric experts in portal hypertension on the management of varices in children. These proceedings follow closely the structure of the workshop. The consensus statements that were agreed upon in each session are reported at the end of the pertinent chapters. The levels of available evidence and the strength of recommendations are graded according to the Oxford System: (http://www.cebm.net/index.aspx?o=1025).

Our deepest thanks go to all the friends who accepted to give lectures and to serve as chairpersons and panellists of the sessions, and who helped us by working hard in the preparation of the workshop and of the chapters.

We also wish to thank Beatrice Rusconi, Gaetano Sabattini, Denise Santi, Anna Maria Sorresso and the entire staff of ADB Eventi e Congressi who managed brilliantly the organization of the workshop, and Sandra Covre, who acted as a consultant in the organization process.

In addition, we are grateful to the European Association for the Study of the Liver (EASL), who supported and endorsed the workshop, and to the following scientific societies who endorsed Baveno V: Associazione Italiana Gastroenterologi ed Endoscopisti Ospedalieri (AIGO), Associazione Italiana per lo Studio del Fegato (AISF), American Society for Gastrointestinal Endoscopy (ASGE), Società Italiana di Endoscopia Digestiva (SIED), Società Italiana di Gastroenterologia (SIGE).

Finally, we wish to thank all the companies who sponsored the workshop, and especially Ferring Pharmaceuticals, who made the publication of this book possible through a generous grant, Phil Boothroyd of Ferring, and Oliver Walter of Blackwell for their encouragement and cooperation in this project, and Blackwell Publishing for the timely and excellent production of this volume.

Roberto de Franchis
On behalf of the Baveno V Scientific Committee

Introduction

Baveno I to Baveno V ... and Beyond

Roberto de Franchis

Department of Medical Sciences, University of Milan, and Gastroenterology 3 Unit, IRCCS Ca' Granda Ospedale Maggiore Policlinico Foundation, Milan, Italy

Since 1986, eight consensus meetings on portal hypertension have been held. The first one was organized by Andrew Burroughs in Groningen, The Netherlands [1]. After Groningen, other meetings followed: in Baveno in 1990 (Baveno I) [2] and 1995 (Baveno II) [3,4], in Milan in 1992 [5], in Reston, USA in 1996 [6], in Stresa in 2000 (Baveno III) [7,8], again in Baveno in 2005 (Baveno IV) [9,10], and in Atlanta, USA in 2007 [11]. This is the ninth meeting of this kind.

The aims of these meetings were to develop definitions of key events in portal hypertension and variceal bleeding, to review the existing evidence on the natural history, the diagnosis and the therapeutic modalities of portal hypertension and to issue evidence-based recommendations for the conduct of clinical trials and the management of patients.

In this review, I will summarize the work previously done in the Baveno workshops I to IV, analyse the impact of the Baveno reports in the medical literature and in clinical practice, and outline what needs to be done in the future.

Baveno I to IV

Topics addressed at the Baveno I–IV workshops

- Definitions of key events
- Diagnostic evaluation of patients with portal hypertension
- Prognostic factors for first bleeding, rebleeding and survival
- Therapeutic strategies in patients with portal hypertension
- Methodological requirements of trials

Attendance at the Baveno workshops

The attendance at the Baveno workshops was 205 participants in Baveno I, 252 in Baveno II, 385 in Baveno III, 485 in Baveno IV and 312 in Baveno V. The proportion of participants from countries outside Italy rose from 19% (Baveno I) to 26% (Baveno II), to 51% (Baveno III), to 62% (Baveno IV) and to 74% (Baveno V). The countries represented were 18 in Baveno I and II, 29 in Baveno III, 40 in Baveno IV and 49 in Baveno V.

Portal Hypertension V, 5th edition. Edited by Roberto de Franchis.
© 2011 Blackwell Publishing Ltd.

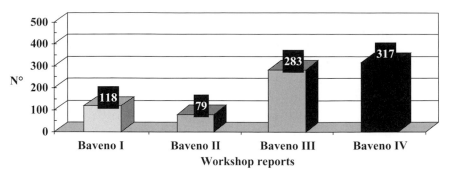

Figure 1 Citations of the Baveno I–IV reports. Total 797 citations as of 17 May 2010.

Publications derived from the Baveno workshops
Reports of the Baveno workshops have been published in the *Journal of Hepatology* in 1992 [2] (Baveno I), in 1996 [3] (Baveno II), in 2000 [7] (Baveno III) and in 2005 [9] (Baveno IV). Proceedings books of the Baveno workshops were published by Blackwell Science in 1996 [4] (Baveno II) and in 2001 [8] (Baveno III), and by Blackwell Publications in 2006 [10] (Baveno IV).

Impact of the Baveno consensus on the medical literature
Figure 1 shows the number of citations of the Baveno I–IV reports in the medical literature between January 1993 and May 2010. Overall, the reports had 797 citations.

Use of the Baveno definitions in clinical trials, 2005–2009
In 12 clinical trials published between 2005 and 2009, on the treatment of acute variceal bleeding, the Baveno definitions of key events (time zero, clinically significant bleeding, failure to control bleeding, rebleeding) have been used in 83.3% of cases.

Application of the Baveno recommendations in clinical practice
Adherence to evidence-based guidelines in clinical practice is an important issue. Over the years, a number of studies have evaluated the application of recommendations issued by different scientific societies in patients with portal hypertension and variceal bleeding. In 2004, Zaman *et al.* [12] evaluated the changes in compliance to the American College of Gastroenterology guidelines between 1997 and 2000. Endoscopic screening of patients to detect oesophageal varices increased from 18% to 54% (p < 0.005). Use of vasoactive drugs prior to endoscopy in suspected variceal bleeders increased from 56% to 83% (p < 0.005). In 2007, Charpignon *et al.* [13] evaluated the impact of a consensus workshop on portal hypertension organized by the French Association for the Study of the Liver on the management practices in France. Early administration of vasoactive drugs in suspected variceal bleeders increased from 35% in 2003 to 68% in 2004 (p < 0.001); antibiotic

prophylaxis also increased from 61% to 70%, but the difference failed to reach statistical significance ($p = 0.098$). Concerning the Baveno recommendations, a recent study [14] examined the adherence to these recommendations concerning the treatment of acute variceal bleeding and the prevention of rebleeding in a specialized unit compared to a community hospital in two Danish cohorts hospitalized between 2000 and 2007. In acute variceal bleeding, vasoactive drugs were used in 79% in the specialized unit and in 69% in the community hospital ($p = 0.06$); prophylactic antibiotics in 55% and 27% respectively ($p < 0.01$); endoscopic therapy in 86% and 74% respectively ($p = 0.04$). Concerning the prevention of rebleeding, prophylactic treatment was started in 91% of cases in the specialized unit and in 74% in the community hospital ($p < 0.01$), with pharmacological therapy (mainly beta-blockers) being used in 82% and 64% respectively ($p = 0.02$), and endoscopic therapy (band ligation) in 71% and 47% respectively ($p < 0.01$).

Beyond Baveno V
Need for strategies to increase the use of the Baveno definitions in trials and the adherence to the recommendations in clinical practice

Despite the high number of citations of the Baveno reports in the literature, the data shown above indicate that there is ample margin for improvement. The use of the Baveno definitions in trials can be considered as fairly satisfactory. However, some limits in the applicability of these definitions have been pointed out [15] in the past. This suggests that the effort to refine the definitions and to evaluate their applicability in trials should continue.

Although few data exist concerning the overall adherence to the Baveno recommendations in clinical practice, such adherence appears to be fair, at least in specialized units. However, even in this setting, there is a wide margin for improvement, since, for instance, the use of prophylactic antibiotics in variceal bleeders is only 55%. Strategies should be developed to increase the awareness of the recommendations and their application in clinical practice, both by hepatologists and generalists.

Need for young colleagues to take over the task of continuing the Baveno tradition

The Baveno workshops started in 1990, and were held every five years. Therefore, if a Baveno VI is to be organized, it should take place in 2015. Baveno started as the endeavour of a group of friends, all young and enthusiastic, who have kept working hard over the years to ensure its success. However, 20 years have passed, and by the spring of 2015 most of the members of the Baveno V scientific committee will have retired or be near retirement. This means that if the Baveno tradition is to continue, over the next few years younger people sharing the enthusiasm and the dedication of the older ones should step in and be active in the organization of the next Baveno workshop. These people should be able to continue the friendly collaboration that exists among the "Founding Fathers" of Baveno.

Acknowledgements

The Baveno I–V workshops were a concerted effort of the following:

Chairpersons, lecturers, panellists:

Argentina:	J Vorobioff
Austria:	G Krejs
Belgium:	F Nevens
Canada:	J Heathcote, S Ling, N Marcon, G Pomier-Layrargues, I Wanless
Denmark:	U Becker, F Bendtsen, E Christensen, C Gluud, S Møller, TIA Sørensen
Egypt:	G Shiha
France:	B Bernard-Chabert, C Bureau, P Calès, L Castéra, D Lebrec, R Moreau, JP Pascal, C Silvain, D Thabut, D Valla, JP Vinel
Germany:	K Binmøller, W Fleig, G Richter, M Rössle, T Sauerbruch, M Schepke, D Schuppan, M Staritz
UK:	AK Burroughs, E Elias, P Hayes, D Patch, D Westaby
India:	YC Chawla, A Kumar, SK Sarin
Italy:	E Ancona, M Angelico, G Balducci, G Barosi, G Battaglia, M Bolognesi, L. Bolondi, L Cestari, GC Caletti, F Cosentino, G D'Amico, R de Franchis, A Dell'Era,A Gatta, G Gerunda, A Liberati, A Maffei Faccioli, PM Mannucci, C Merkel, M Merli, G Minoli, A Morabito, L Pagliaro, A Peracchia, M Pinzani, M Primignani, O Riggio, P Rossi, C Sabbà, D Sacerdoti, F Salerno, M Senzolo, F Schepis, GP Spina, F Tinè, A Tripodi, V Ziparo, M Zoli
Pakistan:	S Abid
Portugal:	P Alexandrino
Spain:	JG Abraldes, A Albillos, R Bañares, A Berzigotti, J Bosch, A Escorsell, JC García-Pagàn, P Ginés, M Navasa, J Piqué, R Planas, C Ripoll, J Rodès, C Villanueva
Switzerland:	A Hadengue, P Gertsch, C Sieber
Taiwan:	FY Lee, HC Lin, GH Lo
Sweden:	C Søderlund
The Netherlands:	H Janssen, H van Buuren
USA:	A Blei, T Boyer, Chalasani, M Fallon, G Garcia-Tsao, N Grace, R Groszmann, JM Henderson, Y Iwakiri, P Kamath, WR Kim, D Kravetz, L Laine, B Mittman, A Sanyal, V Shah, B Shneider, J Talwalkar, G van Stiegmann

Organization:
S Covre, ADB Eventi e Congressi (Beatrice Rusconi, Gaetano Sabattini, Denise Santi, Anna Maria Sorresso)

References

1. Burroughs AK (ed.) (1987) *Methodology and review of clinical trials in portal hypertension.* Excerpta Medical Congress Service No. 763: Amsterdam, New York, Oxford.

2. de Franchis R, Pascal JP, Ancona E, *et al.* (1992) Definitions, methodology and therapeutic strategies in portal hypertension. A consensus development workshop. *J Hepatol* **15**:256–61.

3. de Franchis R (1996) Developing consensus in portal hypertension. *J Hepatol* **25**:390–4.

4. de Franchis R (1996) *Portal Hypertension II. Proceedings of the Second Baveno International Consensus Workshop on Definitions, Methodology and Therapeutic Strategies.* Blackwell Science: Oxford.

5. Spina GP, Arcidiacono R, Bosch J, *et al.* (1994) Gastric endoscopic features in portal hypertension: final report of a consensus conference. *J Hepatol* **21**:461–7.

6. Grace ND, Groszmann RJ, Garcia-Tsao G, *et al.* (1998) Portal hypertension and variceal bleeding: an AASLD single-topic symposium. *Hepatology* **28**:868–80.

7. de Franchis R (2000) Updating consensus in portal hypertension. Report of the Baveno III consensus workshop on definitions, methodology and therapeutic strategies in portal hypertension. *J Hepatol* **33**:846–52.

8. de Franchis R (2000) *Portal Hypertension III. Proceedings of the Third Baveno International Consensus Workshop on Definitions, Methodology and Therapeutic Strategies.* Blackwell Science: Oxford.

9. de Franchis R (2005) Evolving consensus in portal hypertension. *J Hepatol* **43**:167–76.

10. de Franchis R (2006) *Portal Hypertension IV. Proceedings of the Fourth Baveno International Consensus Workshop on Methodology of Diagnosis and Treatment.* Blackwell Publishing: Oxford.

11. Garcia-Tsao G, Bosch J, Groszmann R (2008) Portal hypertension and variceal bleeding, unresolved issues. Summary of an American Association for the Study of Liver Disease and European Association for the Study of the Liver single-topic conference. *Hepatology* **47**:1764–72.

12. Zaman A, Hapke RJ, Flora K, Rosen HR, Benner KG (2004) Changing compliance to the American College of Gastroenterology guidelines for the management of variceal hemorrhage. *Am J Gastroenterol* **99**:645–9.

13. Charpignon C, Oberti F, Bernard P, *et al.* (2007) Management practices for gastrointestinal hemorrhage related to portal hypertension in cirrhotic patients: evaluation of the impact of the Paris consensus workshop. *Gastroenterol Clin Biol* **31**:970–4.

14. Hobolth L, Krag A, Malchow-Moeller A, *et al.* (2010) Adherence to guidelines in bleeding esophageal varices and effects on outcome: comparison between a specialized unit and a community hospital. *Eur J Gastroenterol Hepatol*, in press.

15. Calès P, Lacave N, Silvain C, *et al.* (2000) Prospective study of the application of the Baveno II Consensus Conference criteria in patients with cirrhosis and gastrointestinal bleeding. *J Hepatol* **33**:738–41.

Lecture 6

Pre-primary and Primary Prophylaxis: What Has Been Done?

Carlo Merkel[1], Manuela Merli[2] and Alessandra Dell'Era[3]

[1] Hepatic Haemodynamic Laboratory and Clinica Medica 5, Department of Clinical and Experimental Medicine, University of Padua, Padova, Italy
[2] Division of Gastroenterology, Department of Clinical Medicine, University of Rome "La Sapienza", Rome, Italy
[3] Department of Medical Sciences, Università degli Studi di Milano, IRCCS Ca' Granda Ospedale Maggiore Policlinico Foundation, Milan, Italy

Introduction

The history of treatment of portal hypertension is characterized by an initial phase, during which only patients with the most severe conditions were selected for treatment, followed by a progressive trend towards treatment of earlier stages and less risky conditions. Medical treatment of portal hypertension started in the 1950s, when vasopressin was introduced for treatment of acute variceal bleeding. This was followed by the demonstration of the usefulness of non-selective beta-blockers (NSBB) in the prevention of re-bleeding [1], the prevention of first variceal bleeding in patients with large varices [2] and, more recently, also in patients with small varices [3]. Prevention of varices formation is not a clinical indication for medical treatment as yet but remains a fascinating area of research that is likely to be explored further over the next few years.

This chapter is an overview of treatment of portal hypertension in primary and pre-primary prophylaxis over the past 20 years, from the point of view of the Baveno consensus conferences, which have been held at five-year intervals, starting from 1990.

Pre-primary prophylaxis in portal hypertension

The subject of pre-primary prophylaxis, that is, a treatment aimed at avoiding/delaying the formation of oesophageal varices, was not addressed at Baveno I (1990) [4] or II (1995) [5]. At the time, there was general agreement that NSBB were indicated in the treatment of portal hypertension in patients with large varices, while the usefulness of treating patients with small or no varices remained debated due to insufficient data.

Pre-primary prophylaxis came to the fore at Baveno III (2000) [6] and IV (2005) [7] and Baveno III introduced a new chapter on pre-primary prophylaxis. A number of pathophysiological aspects were discussed, suggesting that factors other than portal hypertension might be involved in the opening of new collaterals, namely modulation of the vascular tone in portal-systemic collaterals and possibly neo-vascularization. These new pathophysiological data lent support to the working hypothesis that introducing treatment at an early stage (small or no varices) might be of benefit.

The appropriateness of starting prophylaxis of variceal bleeding in patients with small oesophageal varices at low risk of bleeding was defined as an interesting area of investigation. At the time, only two studies were available on the topic: one in full [8] and the other one as an interim analysis [9]. In addition, the results appeared controversial. The study by Calés and coworkers [8] reported a larger incidence of variceal size increase in patients treated with NSBB compared to those treated with placebo after one year. The interim analysis in the study by Merkel and coworkers [9] showed a trend towards a decreased progression of varices in patients treated with nadolol vs. placebo. No data were available on the effect of medical treatment in preventing the occurrence of oesophageal varices.

At Baveno IV (2005) the field of pre-primary prophylaxis was discussed in more depth. From a pathophysiological point of view, evidence was arising that the increase in portal pressure causes an up-regulation in endothelial NO synthase (eNOS) in the arterial splanchnic circulation and, in turn, an increase in NO production in experimental models of portal hypertension. Collateral formation was ascribed to a dynamic interplay between vasodilation, vascular remodelling and neo-angiogenesis.

In the clinical setting, the natural history of oesophageal varices formation was subject to further investigation. It appeared that cirrhotic patients without varices developed new varices at a rate of 5–10% per year. The rate of progression from small to medium-large varices ranged from 5 to 20% per year. Alcohol misuse and worsening liver dysfunction were found to accelerate the rate of progression, while abstinence from alcohol seemed to induce varices regression, at least in a subset of patients. The role of non-variceal collateral shunts was also examined, and it was concluded that these do not protect from oesophageal varices formation, rather they are a parallel event reflecting the progression of portal hypertension itself.

Categories of patients in whom pre-primary prophylaxis was worth considering were defined: patients with HVPG 6–10 mmHg and no varices, patients with HVPG > 10 mmHg and no varices and patients with small oesophageal varices (although the last category was also included within the primary prophylaxis setting).

Information on pre-primary prophylaxis was derived from three studies [3,8,10], which considered patients with no varices, small varices, or a combination of the two. The first study [8], on 206 cirrhotic patients with cirrhosis (mostly alcohol-related) and small or no varices, failed to find a protective effect of propranolol in relation to the development of large varices. At two years, large varices were more frequent in the treatment group compared to the placebo group, although the difference was no longer statistically significant at three years of follow-up. The study had a high drop-out rate and the potential influence of abstinence from alcohol was not analysed. The multicentre RCT by Groszmann et al. [10] randomized 213 patients with cirrhosis, no varices and HVPG > 6 mmHg for a NSBB (timolol) or placebo. More than 60% of these patients had HVPG > 10 mmHg, although varices had not appeared yet. Treatment with a NSBB was unable to prevent variceal formation and was associated with a high proportion of adverse events requiring withdrawal from treatment or dose reduction (50% of patients). Treatment was discontinued prematurely in 18% of patients while a further 20% were non-compliant to treatment. In the third study, 161 cirrhotic patients with small varices were randomized to NSBB or placebo [3]. Patients receiving the NSBB showed a significant reduction of the risk of variceal enlargement and variceal bleeding, associated with a modest decrease in HVPG, which was measured in a subset.

The working group debated the meaning of these results: collateral circulation was interpreted as a consequence of portal hypertension and hyperdynamic circulation. NSBB were expected to act as vasoconstrictors on the portal venous system, including collateral circulation. Patients with portal hypertension and no varices were regarded as those in whom haemodynamic changes were less pronounced; hence, the lack of efficacy of NSBB in these patients. In contrast, in patients with small varices haemodynamic changes were thought to be fully developed. Thus these patients were expected to respond to NSBB. The panel concluded that there was no indication to treat cirrhotic patients with NSBB to prevent the formation of varices. Whether NSBB could be used to prevent progression of small varices could not be ascertained due to limited data. Subsequent guidelines considered NSBB adequate for use in patients with small varices.

Primary prophylaxis of variceal bleeding

In patients with cirrhosis and oesophageal varices, the incidence of first variceal bleeding ranges from 12% to 15% per year [11]. In spite of all the improvements made in the setting of acute variceal bleeding treatment, the mortality rate is still high, at approximately 15–20% [11]. Therefore, the prevention of the first variceal bleed is mandatory. The main factors predicting the risk of variceal bleeding are variceal size, red wale marks on the variceal wall and the degree of liver dysfunction [12]. These epidemiological data are the basis for the clinical recommendation that patients at high risk of bleeding from oesophageal varices should start primary prophylaxis [4–7].

The recommendation of Baveno II and III [5, 6] was to start prophylaxis of first variceal bleeding in all patients with high-risk varices, considering that endoscopic criteria have the highest value in defining the risk of bleeding, even though other criteria (i.e. liver function, aetiology of cirrhosis) might also be important. At the time, only patients with large varices were considered candidates for treatment. The recommended therapy was with NSBB, namely, propranolol or nadolol.

At Baveno III, the experts focused their attention on the methods required to monitor beta-blockade [7]. In clinical practice, the dose of NSBB is generally increased stepwise with the target of achieving a 25% reduction in resting heart rate or until reaching a resting heart rate of 55 bpm, or until the development of symptoms. It appeared that some patients treated with NSBB achieving these targets were still not protected from variceal bleeding. It was emphasized that there was no relationship between the degree of beta-blockade, as assessed by the reduction in resting heart rate, and the reduction in portal pressure or protection from variceal bleeding.

Changes in HVPG during treatment were defined as the only index that discriminates between patients treated with NSBB who are actually protected from variceal bleeding (good responders) from those who are not (poor responders). Good responders were defined as those reaching a reduction in HVPG below 12 mmHg or more than 20% from baseline [13,14]. However, since the risk of bleeding in primary prophylaxis is 12–15% per year, it was not surprising that about 60% of patients treated with NSBB who did not achieve these targets would not bleed in a two-year follow-up [14]. In the Baveno IV consensus statement, it was agreed that HVPG monitoring identifies patients with cirrhosis who will benefit from NSBB therapy in primary prophylaxis, that "a la carte" treatment using HVPG response in primary prophylaxis needed to be evaluated, especially in high-risk patients, but also that until then routine use of HVPG could not be recommended. It was also agreed that there is no indication to endoscopic follow-up of patients on pharmacological therapy.

The effect of NSBB in reducing the incidence of first variceal bleeding was studied in a series of randomized clinical trials [15], in which NSSB reduced the bleeding rate from approximately 25% to 15% in a two-year median follow-up. A Cochrane meta-analysis performed in 2004 showed that NSBB also produce a significant reduction in mortality [16]. At the Baveno IV consensus conference, the indication for primary prophylaxis with NSBB in patients with medium-large varices was confirmed, and also extended to patients with small varices, even though it was stated that further studies were required before a formal recommendation on the latter could be made. Patients with small varices with red wale signs or belonging to Child class C were also considered suitable for treatment, because of their increased risk of bleeding.

In the past 20 years a series of other pharmacological agents have been tested in the setting of primary prophylaxis. Isosorbide-5-mononitrate (ISMN) in monotherapy was at first considered an option for patients with contraindication or intolerance to NSBB [5]. However, subsequent studies [17–19] led the Baveno IV experts to state that the use of ISMN alone was not recommended because of lack of efficacy in patients with large varices, and increased risk of death in older patients. The association of ISMN with NSBB has been evaluated in a long-term study in which it was shown to reduce the rate of first bleeding episodes without effects on mortality [20,21]. However, two subsequent RCTs failed to confirm these positive results and showed an increase in side-effects [22,23]. At Baveno III and IV it was stated that there is not enough data to recommend the use of a combination of NSBB and nitrates [6,7]. Similarly, there was insufficient evidence to suggest the use of spironolactone in association with NSBB [24].

Other drugs are currently under evaluation for primary prophylaxis, to include carvedilol (a NSBB with vasodilating properties), which is particularly promising. Indeed, a recent RCT comparing carvedilol with endoscopic variceal ligation (EVL) showed that this drug was associated with lower variceal bleeding and adverse event rate than EVL, without significant differences in mortality [25].

From Baveno II (1995) [5] onwards, endoscopic techniques were also taken into consideration for purposes of primary prophylaxis. In that meeting it was stated that endoscopic sclerotherapy should not be used in primary prophylaxis because of lack of efficacy and increased mortality rate [5,26–28], and that new endoscopic therapies such as EVL had not been established as a prophylactic measure to prevent variceal bleeding. At Baveno III (2000) [6], data on EVL in primary prophylaxis were considered encouraging in high-risk patients, but too preliminary to lead to a formal statement. In 2005, two meta-analyses [29, 30] demonstrated that EVL, compared to NSBB, is associated with lower incidence of first variceal bleeding without differences in mortality. Thus, at Baveno IV it was stated that NSBB decrease the risk of first variceal bleeding, and that prophylactic EVL is useful in preventing variceal bleeding in patients with medium and large oesophageal varices [7]. It was also highlighted that the long-term benefits of EVL were uncertain because of the short duration of follow-up. A subsequent meta-analysis showed that the positive effect of EVL might depend on the duration of follow-up (i.e. the shorter the follow-up, the better the effect) and that EVL and NSBB are probably equally as effective [31].

Over the years, increasing attention was devoted to patients with large oesophageal varices with contraindications or intolerance to NSBB (both groups of approximately 15% of patients). At Baveno III [6] no consensus was reached about the treatment of these patients because of the lack of studies addressing the issue. It was stated that preliminary data suggested that ISMN is not a good option and that EVL might be useful. At Baveno IV [7] it was stated that EVL should be offered to patients with medium–large varices and contraindications or intolerance to NSBB.

Conclusions

Looking back at the past 20 years, it appears that our understanding of the mechanisms involved in the development of portal hypertension and our management strategies in the primary prophylaxis setting have changed to a considerable extent. We hope that the next 20 years will be at least as fruitful, if not more.

References

1. Lebrec D, Nouel O, Corbic M, *et al.* (1980) Propranolol – a medical treatment for portal hypertension? *Lancet* **2**:180–2.
2. Pascal JP, Calès P, Multicenter Study Group (1987) Propranolol in the prevention of first upper digestive tract hemorrhage in patients with cirrhosis of the liver and esophageal varices. *N Engl J Med* **317**:856–61.
3. Merkel C, Marin R, Angeli P, *et al.* (2004) A placebo-controlled clinical trial of nadolol in the prophylaxis of growth of small esophageal varices in cirrhosis. *Gastroenterology* **127**:476–84.

4. de Franchis R, Pascal JP, Ancona E, *et al.* (1992) Definitions, methodology and therapeutic strategies in portal hypertension. A consensus development workshop. *J Hepatol* **15**:256–61.

5. de Franchis R (1996) Developing consensus in portal hypertension. *J Hepatol* **25**:390–4.

6. de Franchis R (2000) Updating consensus in portal hypertension. Report of the Baveno III consensus workshop on definitions, methodology and therapeutic strategies in portal hypertension. *J Hepatol* **33**:846–85.

7. de Franchis R (2005) Evolving consensus in portal hypertension. Report of the Baveno IV consensus workshop on methodology of diagnosis and therapy in portal hypertension. *J Hepatol* **43**:167–76.

8. Calés P, Oberti F, Payen JL, *et al.* (1999) Lack of effect of propranolol in the prevention of large esophageal varices in patients with cirrhosis: a randomized trial. *Eur J Gastroenterol Hepatol* **11**:741–5.

9. Merkel C, Angeli P, Marin R, *et al.* (1998) Beta-blockers in the prevention of aggravation of esophageal varices in patients with cirrhosis and small esophageal varices: interim analysis of a controlled clinical trial. *Hepatology* **28** (Suppl 1): 453A (abstract).

10. Groszmann RJ, Garcia-Tsao G, Bosch J, *et al.* (2005) Beta-blockers to prevent gastroesophageal varices in patients with cirrhosis. *N Engl J Med*, **353**:2254–61.

11. Garcia-Tsao G, Lim J, Members of the Veterans Affairs Hepatitis C Resource Center Program (2009) Management and treatment of patients with cirrhosis and portal hypertension: recommendations from the Department of Veterans Affairs Hepatitis C Resource Center Program and the National Hepatitis C Program. *Am J Gastroenterol* **104**:1802–29.

12. North Italian Endoscopic Club for the Study and Treatment of Esophageal Varices (1988) Prediction of the first variceal hemorrhage in patients with cirrhosis of the liver and esophageal varices. A prospective multicenter study. *N Engl J Med* **319**:983–9.

13. Groszmann RJ, Bosch J, Grace ND, *et al.* (1990) Hemodynamic events in a prospective randomized trial of propranolol versus placebo in the prevention of a first variceal hemorrhage. *Gastroenterology* **99**:1401–7.

14. Feu F, Garcia Pagan JC, Bosch J, *et al.* (1995) Relation between portal pressure response to pharmacotherapy and risk of recurrent variceal haemorrhage in patients with cirrhosis. *Lancet* **346**:1056–9.

15. D'Amico G, Pagliaro L, Bosch J (1999) Pharmacological treatment of portal hypertension: an evidence-based approach. *Semin Liv Dis* **19**:475–505.

16. Chen W, Nikolova D, Frederiksen SL, *et al.* (2004) Beta-blockers reduce mortality in cirrhotic patients with oesophageal varices who have never bled (Cochrane review). *J Hepatol* **40**:67 (abstract).

17. Garcia-Pagan JC, Villanueva C, Vila MC, *et al.* (2001) Isosorbide mononitrate in the prevention of first variceal bleed in patients who cannot receive beta-blockers. *Gastroenterology* **121**:908–14.

18. Borroni G, Salerno F, Cazzaniga M, *et al.* (2002) Nadolol is superior to isosorbide mononitrate for the prevention of the first variceal bleeding in cirrhotic patients with ascites. *J Hepatol* **37**:315–21.

19. Angelico M, Carli L, Piat C, *et al.* (1997) Effects of isosorbide-5-mononitrate compared with propranolol on first bleeding and long-term survival in cirrhosis. *Gastroenterology* **113**:1632–9.

20. Merkel C, Marin R, Enzo E, *et al.* (1996) Randomised trial of nadolol alone or with isosorbide mononitrate for primary prophylaxis of variceal bleeding in cirrhosis. Gruppo-Triveneto per L'ipertensione portale (GTIP). *Lancet* **348**:1677–81.

21. Merkel C, Marin R, Sacerdoti D, *et al.* (2000) Long-term results of a clinical trial of nadolol with or without isosorbide mononitrate for primary prophylaxis of variceal bleeding in cirrhosis. *Hepatology* **31**:324–9.
22. Garcia-Pagan JC, Morillas R, Banares R, *et al.* (2003) Propranolol plus placebo versus propranolol plus isosorbide-5-mononitrate in the prevention of a first variceal bleed: a double-blind RCT. *Hepatology* **37**:1260–6.
23. D'Amico G, Pasta L, Politi F, *et al.* (2002) Isosorbide mononitrate with nadolol compared to nadolol alone for prevention of the first bleeding in cirrhosis. A double-blind placebo-controlled randomized trial. *Gastroenterol Int* **15**:40–5.
24. Abecasis R, Kravetz D, Fassio E, *et al.* (2003) Nadolol plus spironolactone in the prophylaxis of first variceal bleed in non ascitic cirrhotic patients: a preliminary study. *Hepatology* **37**:359–65.
25. Tripathi D, Ferguson JW, Kochar N, *et al.* (2009) Randomized controlled trial of carvedilol versus variceal band ligation for the prevention of the first variceal bleed. *Hepatology* **50**:825–33.
26. D'Amico G, Pagliaro L, Bosch J (1995) The treatment of portal hypertension: a meta-analytic review. *Hepatology* **22**:332–54.
27. Pagliaro L, D'Amico G, Sorensen TIA, *et al.* (1997) Prevention of first bleeding in cirrhosis. A meta-analysis of randomized clinical trials of non-surgical treatment. *Ann Intern Med* **17**:59–70.
28. Veterans Affairs Cooperative Variceal Sclerotherapy Group (1991) Prophylactic sclerotherapy for esophageal varices in men with alcoholic liver disease. A randomized, single-blind, multicenter clinical trial. *N Engl J Med* **324**:1779–84.
29. Khuroo MS, Khuroo NS, Farahat KL, *et al.* (2005) Meta-analysis: endoscopic variceal ligation for primary prophylaxis of oesophageal variceal bleeding. *Aliment Pharmacol Ther* **21**:347–61.
30. Garcia-Pagan JC, Bosch J (2005) Endoscopic band ligation in the treatment of portal hypertension. *Nat Clin Pract Gastroenterol Hepatol* **2**:526–35.
31. Gluud LL, Klingenberg S, Nikolova D, *et al.* (2007) Banding ligation versus beta-blockers as primary prophylaxis in esophageal varices: systematic review of randomized trials. *Am J Gastroenterol* **102**:2842–8.

Lecture 7

Pre-Primary and Primary Prophylaxis: What Should We Do Next?

Roberto J Groszmann[1], Cristina Ripoll[2] and Julio Vorobioff[3]

[1]Yale University School of Medicine, New Haven, CT, and VA and CT Healthcare System, Digestive Diseases Section, West Haven, CT, USA

[2]Hepatology and Liver Transplant Unit, Digestive Diseases Department, Hospital General Universitario Gregorio Marañón, Centro de Investigación Biomédica en Red de Enfermedades Hepáticas y Digestivas (CIBERehd), Madrid, Spain

[3]University of Rosario Medical School, Rosario, Argentina

Introduction

In the previous chapter we have already discussed what has been done in the area of pre-primary and primary prophylaxis of variceal bleeding. We would like now to propose what areas we believe require additional studies.

Pre-primary prophylaxis

During the last Baveno consensus meeting (Baveno IV) it was stated that "*there is no indication, at this time, to treat patients to prevent the formation of varices*" [1] and at the more recent AASLD-EASL meeting it was recommended that, "*unless a new and effective therapy becomes available, further trials of pre-primary prophylaxis with existing therapies are unnecessary*" [2]. Until now the published studies have been designed to evaluate interventions that could prevent or delay the development (if non-existent) or to prevent growth (if already developed, but still small) of oesophageal varices [3,4]. Perhaps, a re-definition of the main objective(s) of pre-primary prophylaxis may be needed before designing new trials. At the aforementioned 2005 Baveno meeting it was concluded that "*patients with small varices could be treated with non-selective β-blockers to prevent progression of varices and bleeding*" and that "*patients with small varices with red wale marks or Child C [5] class have an increased risk of bleeding and may benefit from treatment*". Therefore, this statement included "de facto" small varices in the area of primary prophylaxis [6]. We believe that pre-primary prophylaxis should only include patients *without* gastro-oesophageal varices. The presence of varices in itself places the patient in a different prognostic stage [7]. Prevention in this setting is mainly undertaken to prevent bleeding (and growth in some cases).

Portal Hypertension V, 5th edition. Edited by Roberto de Franchis.
© 2011 Blackwell Publishing Ltd.

The data published in pre-primary prophylaxis to date have not led to encouraging results as the only study [8] that has evaluated the use of non-selective beta-blockers (NSBBs) in the setting of pre-primary prophylaxis had negative results regarding the development of varices. This study included patients with compensated cirrhosis with portal hypertension ($\geq$ 6 mmHg) without varices at baseline. The patients were randomized to placebo or timolol, a NSBB similar to propranolol but 5 to 10 times more potent [9]. The primary endpoint was the development of varices or variceal bleeding while secondary endpoints were the development of ascites, encephalopathy, liver transplantation or death. No differences were detected regarding the primary or secondary endpoint of the study. However, when comparing patients who were randomized to NSBB or placebo, there was a lower incidence of the primary and secondary endpoints during follow-up in those patients (timolol + placebo treated patients) who had a significant >10% decrease in HVPG. Further evaluation of this homogeneous group of compensated cirrhotics identified HVPG, albumin and MELD as independent predictors of decompensation (defined by variceal haemorrhage, ascites, and encephalopathy). An HVPG value of 10 mmHg was identified as the best cutoff, so that patients with a baseline HVPG above this cutoff had an almost six-fold increase in the risk of decompensating during four years follow-up [10]. Perhaps limiting pre-primary prophylactic measures to the patients who are at the greatest risk, that is patients with an HVPG $\geq$ 10 mmHg, would optimize the results.

Patients who have clinically significant portal hypertension ($\geq$ 10 mm Hg), have a more severe hyperdynamic splanchnic circulation with collateralization of the portal system. For this reason, it seems logical that prophylactic efforts, with NSBBs, should be focused mainly on these patients who are at greatest risk. These are the patients who may have the most to benefit from the use of NSBBs and therefore are the ones in which the negative aspects of the side-effects of these drugs could be accepted. On the other hand in patients with mild portal hypertension, treatment should be centred on the source of the increased resistance to portal flow, the liver disease itself, without adding NSBBs or other agents that may reduce portal blood flow. Therefore, risk stratification of patients with mild ($\geq$ 6 $\leq$ 10 mmHg) or clinically significant portal hypertension (10 mmHg) is of utmost importance. Unfortunately, HVPG measurement is a procedure that, although small, does have a minimal risk associated with its invasive nature which precludes its widespread use as many physicians and patients do not consider that the benefit of the measurement overcomes the intrinsic risk. Attempts have been made to identify non-invasive methods to estimate HVPG, or at least to identify those patients with clinically significant portal hypertension. Initial promising results to identify clinically significant portal hypertension with liver stiffness measurement [11], have been encouraging [12, 13]. However, the latter studies included heterogenous populations of patients, both compensated and decompensated so it is difficult to draw clear conclusions from these studies. At any rate it is clear now that a large proportion of patients are not good candidates for this simple test

(BMI > 30) and that some degree of expertise is required before the measurements can be considered reliable [14]. Initial attempts to predict clinically significant portal hypertension with other non-invasive techniques such as ultrasound have not added further information to the one that can be drawn from laboratory tests [15]. Further efforts are necessary in order to establish an appropriate non-invasive method for estimating portal pressure that would allow correct risk stratification. Nevertheless, one thing is to estimate non-invasively HVPG in order to stratify risk and another is to have a precise risk estimation of changes of HVPG that are produced in response to drugs.

In the pre-primary study published in *NEJM* in 2005 [8], the relevant issue seemed to be to achieve a decrease of portal pressure to levels below 10 mmHg or a reduction of at least 10 % from baseline. Then, one may imply that compensated patients may benefit from a decrease in portal pressure independently of the agent used to achieve this aim. Most studies that have evaluated pharmacological reduction of portal pressure in patients have used NSBBs; however it is known that other approaches can reduce portal pressure as well, such as alcohol abstinence or antiviral therapy [16–18]. Although it seems logical to consider that the benefit of the reduction of HVPG will be the same without considering what drug is used to obtain this reduction, there is no scientific evidence to support this hypothesis. In fact, it is possible that HVPG reduction based on decreasing portal venous inflow (propranolol and other beta-blockers) is not the same as HVPG reduction based on a decrease of intrahepatic vascular resistance (simvastatin, interferon, alcohol abstinence, etc). Interestingly, simvastatin improves hepatic fractional and intrinsic clearance of indocyanine green, demonstrating an improvement in effective liver perfusion and function [19], while this has not been the case for beta-blockers [20]. Perhaps, reduction of HVPG by different mechanisms may have a different effect on the incidence of relevant endpoints in patients with cirrhosis.

In summary, it seems that since the presence of clinically significant portal hypertension is associated with the incidence of varices and decompensation, possibly maintaining portal pressure below this level could prevent or delay these events. We should stratify patients according to the degree of portal hypertension, mild and clinically significant. Possibly, in patients with mild portal hypertension ($\geq$ 6 mmHg $\leq$ 10 mmHg) portal hypotensive treatment should be focused on aetiological factors affecting the liver itself while in the case of clinically significant portal hypertension ($\geq$10 mmHg) drugs like NSBBs that act on the hyperdynamic splanchnic circulation may be required on top of the disease-specific treatment. In order to achieve these aims, new and more potent drugs or a combination of drugs that target different implicated factors that cause portal hypertension are necessary.

Primary prophylaxis

The unquestionable beneficial effect of NSBBs in the setting of primary prophylaxis has been discussed already. However, many questions remain to be solved regarding beta-blockers in primary prophylaxis.

A considerable number of physicians use endoscopic variceal ligation as a first approach to prevention of a first variceal bleed. The studies that compared this approach to beta-blockers, overlook the fact that beta-blockers may have other beneficial effects regarding the course of the liver disease itself that are unlikely to be observed with endoscopic variceal ligation. Further studies would be necessary to ascertain the prevention of other complications associated with portal hypertension and end-stage liver disease in those patients who have a favourable haemodynamic response. If this were confirmed, the information derived from the studies comparing the two options should perhaps be reconsidered.

Furthermore, although beta-blockers originate a large number of side-effects, these rarely if ever have induced lethal complications. On the other hand, while endoscopic procedures have a lower incidence of treatments complications, their use has been associated with more serious complications, including death, secondary to bleeding following post-procedure ulcers [5].

Until the present day pre-primary and primary prophylaxis refers to the administration of beta-blockers in order to avoid development of varices or variceal haemorrhage. However, the prognostic relevance of decompensation defined by the presence of variceal haemorrhage, ascites, encephalopathy and jaundice was recently underlined [7]. Patients who remain in the compensated phase of the disease have a median survival over 12 years, while the median survival of patients who are in the decompensated phase is 2 years. Due to the prognostic relevance this event carries, it would be of utmost importance to identify therapeutic options that could postpone or in the best case avoid the onset of decompensation. In this case prophylactic treatment would be used with a different aim, that is, to prevent the development of decompensation.

Several studies have suggested that patients who are on NSBBs and have achieved an appropriate haemodynamic response defined by the decrease of HVPG below the 12 mmHg threshold or at least 20% from baseline have a decrease in the incidence of different complications of end-stage liver disease such as ascites, spontaneous bacterial peritonitis, variceal haemorrhage and hepatorenal syndrome [21–23]. Furthermore this haemodynamic response has been associated with a decrease in mortality [24, 25].

The spectrum of the liver disease in patients in the setting of primary prophylaxis can be wide. Patients with clinically significant portal hypertension and compensated disease may be able to tolerate better carvedilol, a more potent portal hypotensive NSBBs, which can produce arterial hypotension in patients with decompensated disease. Recently an RCT showed that patients who received carvedilol in primary prophylaxis had a lower rate of variceal bleed in comparison to patients who were randomized to endoscopic variceal ligation [26].

Another interesting beta-blocker to explore is nebivolol [27] a beta-blocker that improves endothelial dysfunction via its strong stimulatory effects on the activity of the endothelial nitric oxide synthase and via its antioxidative properties. Because impaired endothelial activity is attributed an important causal role in the pathophysiology of intrahepatic portal hypertension, the endothelium-agonistic properties of nebivolol suggest that this drug might provide additional benefit beyond beta-receptor blockade. It would be interesting to explore the effect of this drug, which has a very weak vasoconstrictive effect because it lacks beta-2 adrenergic blocker properties, in patients with mild portal hypertension in whom increase in intrahepatic vascular resistance plays the major role in maintaining portal hypertension.

Great discrepancy in the management of beta-blockers has been observed among experts. Given that most studies exclude patients with associated comorbidities (e.g. Chronic Obstructive Pulmonary Disease (COPD), Congestive Heart Failure (CHF)), our current experience with NSBB in these settings is smaller; however, possibly compensated patients may tolerate better the third generation of beta-blockers such as carvedilol or nebivolol. In the setting of cardiovascular disease, beta-blockers, particularly carvedilol, are an important pillar of the prevention and treatment of heart failure [28] and should therefore not be withdrawn due to this comorbidity. Nebivolol is also much better tolerated in the setting of COPD. The use of beta-blockers in the setting of advanced liver disease with circulatory dysfunction including patients with refractory ascites, type 2 hepatorenal syndrome and cirrhotic cardiomyopathy remains to be determined.

In the last decade the aetiological factors leading to a hyperdynamic splanchnic circulation have been clarified. Therefore, it is likely that future treatments for preventing the complications of portal hypertension will include not only the classical beta-blockers and treatment of the primary liver disease itself but also treatments specifically directed at preventing or ameliorating the hyperdynamic state.

Lastly it will be of great interest to unravel the mechanism of NSBB failure since it is possible that the reasons leading to NSBB failure could be applied also to other compounds that reduce portal pressure by similar mechanisms. During chronic treatment of portal hypertension with NSBB, responders (i.e. patients in whom HVPG decreases to ≤ 12 mmHg or $\geq 20\%$ from baseline value) account for approximately 40% of the patients. This group of patients have a significant reduction of portal hypertensive-related complications [21–23] and an improved survival [24, 25]. Whether this finding can be enhanced by increasing the number of patients who achieve a favourable haemodynamic response remains to be determined. Increasing the number of patients who achieve a favourable haemodynamic response can be accomplished by new therapeutic options or a redefinition of the favourable haemodynamic response. A smaller reduction (i.e. 10%) of HVPG in repeat (chronic) measurement has also been shown to be relevant regarding the incidence of first variceal bleed [29] with an increase in specificity and only a slight reduction of sensitivity. By reducing the necessary decrease to define responders, one decreases the grey zone [30] of non-responders who do not bleed during follow-up and therefore can more adequately define the population of non-responders who are at risk of bleeding and perhaps need other therapeutic options.

If we redefine the concept of pre-primary and/or primary prophylaxis to a broader definition it would be possible to unify the concept of prophylaxis into a single aim, namely to prevent decompensation.

References

1. Groszmann RJ, Merkel C, Iwakiri Y, *et al.* (2006) Prevention of the formation of varices (pre-primary prophylaxis). In: de Franchis R (ed.) *Portal Hypertension IV. Proceedings of the Fourth Baveno International Consensus Workshop on Definitions, Methodology and Therapeutic Strategies.* Blackwell Science: Oxford, pp. 103–151.

2. Garcia-Tsao G, Bosch J, Groszmann RJ (2008) Portal hypertension and variceal bleeding – unresolved issues. Summary of an American Association for the Study of Liver Diseases and European Association for the Study of the Liver single-topic conference. *Hepatology* **44**:1764–72.

3. Merkel C, Marin R, Angeli P, *et al.* (2004) A placebo-controlled clinical trial of nadolol in the prophylaxis of growth of small esophageal varices in cirrhosis. *Gastroenterology* **127**:476–84.

4. Calès P, Oberti F, Payen JL, *et al.* (1999) Lack of effect of propranolol in the prevention of large oesophageal varices in patients with cirrhosis: a randomized trial. *Eur J Gastroenterol Hepatol* **11**:741–5.

5. Garcia-Tsao G, Bosch J (2010) Management of varices and variceal hemorrhage. *N Engl J Med* **362**:823–32.

6. Grace N, García-Pagan JC, Angelico M, *et al.* (2006) Primary prophylaxis for variceal bleeding. In: de Franchis R (ed.) *Portal Hypertension IV. Proceedings of the Fourth Baveno International Consensus Workshop on Definitions, Methodology and Therapeutic Strategies.* Blackwell Science: Oxford, pp. 168–200.

7. D'Amico G, Garcia-Tsao G, Pagliaro L (2006) Natural history and prognostic indicators of survival in cirrhosis: a systematic review of 118 studies. *J Hepatol* **44**:217–31.

8. Groszmann RJ, Garcia-Tsao G, Bosch J, *et al.* (2005) Beta-blockers to prevent gastroesophageal varices in patients with cirrhosis. *N Engl J Med* **353**:2254–61.

9. Weiner N (1980) Drugs that inhibit adrenergic nerves and block adrenergic receptors. In: Goodman Gilman A, Goodman LS, Gilman A (eds) *Goodman and Gilman's The Pharmacological Basis of Therapeutics* (6th ed.). Macmillan: New York, pp. 176–210.

10. Ripoll C, Groszmann R, Garcia-Tsao G, *et al.* (2007) Hepatic venous pressure gradient predicts clinical decompensation in patients with compensated cirrhosis. *Gastroenterology* **133**:481–8.

11. Vizzutti F, Arena U, Romanelli RG, *et al.* (2007) Liver stiffness measurement predicts severe portal hypertension in patients with HCV-related cirrhosis. *Hepatology* **45**:1290–7.

12. Bureau C, Metivier S, Peron JM, *et al.* (2008) Transient elastography accurately predicts presence of significant portal hypertension in patients with chronic liver disease. *Aliment Pharmacol Ther* **27**:1261–8.

13. Lemoine M, Katsahian S, Ziol M *et al.* (2008) Liver stiffness measurement as a predictive tool of clinically significant portal hypertension in patients with compensated hepatitis C virus or alcohol-related cirrhosis. *Aliment Pharmacol Ther* **28**:1102–10.

14. Castéra L, Foucher J, Bernard PH, *et al.* (2010) Pitfalls of liver stiffness measurement: A 5-year prospective study of 13,369 examinations. *Hepatology* **51**:828–35.

15. Berzigotti A, Gilabert R, Abraldes JG, *et al.* (2008) Noninvasive prediction of clinically significant portal hypertension and esophageal varices in patients with compensated liver cirrhosis. *Am J Gastroenterol* **103**:1159–67.

16. Vorobioff J, Groszmann RJ, Picabea E, *et al.* (1996) Prognostic value of hepatic venous pressure gradient measurements in alcoholic cirrhosis: a 10-year prospective study. *Gastroenterology* **111**:701–9.

17. Rincon D, Ripoll C, Lo Iacono O, *et al.* (2006) Antiviral therapy decreases hepatic venous pressure gradient in patients with chronic hepatitis C and advanced fibrosis. *Am J Gastroenterol* **101**:2269–74.

18. Manolakopoulos S, Triantos C, Theodoropoulos J, *et al.* (2009) Antiviral therapy reduces portal pressure in patients with cirrhosis due to HBeAg-negative chronic hepatitis B and significant portal hypertension. *J Hepatol* **51**:468–74.

19. Abraldes JG, Albillos A, Bañares R, *et al.* (2009) Simvastatin lowers portal pressure in patients with cirrhosis and portal hypertension: a randomized controlled trial. *Gastroenterology* **136**:1651–8.

20. Bendtsen F, Henriksen JH, Becker U, *et al.* (1987) Effect of oral propranolol on splanchnic oxygen uptake and haemodynamics in patients with cirrhosis. *J Hepatol* **5**:137–43

21. Turnes J, Garcia-Pagan JC, Abraldes JG, *et al.* (2006) Pharmacological reduction of portal pressure and long-term risk of first variceal bleeding in patients with cirrhosis. *Am J Gastroenterol* **101**:506–12.

22. Villanueva C, Lopez-Balaguer JM, Aracil C, *et al.* (2004) Maintenance of hemodynamic response to treatment for portal hypertension and influence on complications of cirrhosis. *J Hepatol* **40**:757–65.

23. Abraldes JG, Tarantino I, Turnes J, *et al.* (2003) Hemodynamic response to pharmacological treatment of portal hypertension and long-term prognosis of cirrhosis. *Hepatology* **37**:902–8.

24. Groszmann RJ, Bosch J, Grace N, *et al.* (1990) Hemodynamic events in a prospective randomized trial of propranolol vs. placebo in the prevention of a first variceal hemorrhage. *Gastroenterology* **99**:1401–7.

25. Albillos A, Banares R, González M, *et al.* (2007) Value of the hepatic venous pressure gradient to monitor drug therapy for portal hypertension: a meta-analysis. *Am J Gastroenterology* **102**:1116–26.

26. Tripathi D, Ferguson JW, Kochar N, *et al.* (2009) Randomized controlled trial of carvedilol versus variceal band ligation for the prevention of the first variceal bleed. *Hepatology* **50**:825–33.

27. Munzel T, Gori T (2009) Nebivolol: the somewhat-different beta-adrenergic receptor blocker. *J Am Coll Cardiol* **54**:1491–9.

28. Klapholz M (2009) Beta-blocker use for the stages of heart failure. *Mayo Clin Proc* **84**:718–29.

29. Villanueva C, Aracil C, Colomo A, *et al.* (2009) Acute hemodynamic response to beta-blockers and prediction of long-term outcome in primary prophylaxis of variceal bleeding. *Gastroenterology* **137**:119–28.

30. Thalheimer U, Bosch J, Patch D, Burroughs A (2008) Improved survival with nonselective beta blockers. *Hepatology* **48**:2091–2.

Baveno V Consensus Statements

Pre-primary and Primary Prophylaxis

Roberto Groszmann, Carlo Merkel (Chairperson), Alessandra Dell'Era, Manuela Merli, Cristina Ripoll and Julio Vorobioff

Pre-primary prophylaxis (prevention of the formation of varices)

Background

- Prevention of the development of complications of portal hypertension is an important area of research. (5;D)
- Hepatic venous pressure gradient (HVPG) ≥ 10 mmHg is predictive of varices formation and decompensation. (1b;A)

Recommendations for management

- Pre-primary prophylaxis should only include patients without gastro-oesophageal varices. (5;D)
- All cirrhotic patients should be screened for varices at diagnosis.
- Treatment of underlying liver disease may reduce portal hypertension and prevent its clinical complications. (1b;A)
- There is no indication, at this time, to use beta-blockers to prevent the formation of varices. (1b;A)
- HVPG measurement in pre-primary prophylaxis may be recommended only in the context of clinical trials. (5;D)

Areas requiring further study

- Basic mechanisms in the development and progression of portal hypertension.
- Non-invasive techniques to identify patients with clinically significant portal hypertension.
- The impact of treating the underlying chronic liver disease in the development of varices and other portal hypertensive-related complications.
- Treatments to prevent the development of varices and other portal hypertensive-related complications in different risk groups (e.g. patients with HVPG between 6–10 mmHg and those with HVPG ≥10 mmHg).

Portal Hypertension V, 5th edition. Edited by Roberto de Franchis.
© 2011 Blackwell Publishing Ltd.

Prevention of the first bleeding episode
Patients with small varices
- Patients with small varices with red wale marks or Child C class have an increased risk of bleeding (1b; A) and should be treated with non-selective beta-blockers (NSBB). (5;D)
- Patients with small varices without signs of increased risk may be treated with NSBB to prevent progression of varices and bleeding. (1b;A) Further studies are required to confirm their benefit.

Patients with medium–large varices
- Either NSBB or endoscopic band ligation (EBL) is recommended for the prevention of first variceal bleeding of medium or large varices. (1a;A)
- Choice of treatment should be based on local resources and expertise, patient preference and characteristics, side-effects and contraindications. (5;D)
- Carvedilol is a promising alternative (1b;A) that needs to be further explored.
- Shunt therapy, endoscopic sclerotherapy, and isosorbide mononitrate alone should not be used in the prophylaxis of first variceal bleeding. (1a;A)
- There is insufficient data to recommend the use of NSBB in combination with isosorbide-5-mononitrate (ISMN), spironolactone, or EBL for primary prophylaxis. (1b;A)

Patients with gastric varices
- Despite the absence of specific data on prophylactic studies, patients with gastric varices may be treated with NSBB. (5;D)

Role of HVPG measurement
- In centres where adequate resources and expertise are available, HVPG measurements should be routinely used for prognostic and therapeutic indications. (5;D)
- Controlled trials using pharmacological therapy in primary prophylaxis should include HVPG measurements. (5;D)
- A decrease in HVPG of at least 20% from baseline or to ≤ 12 mmHg after chronic treatment with NSBB is clinically relevant in the setting of primary prophylaxis. (1a;A)
- Acute HVPG response to intravenous propranolol may be used to identify responders to beta-blockers; specifically a decrease in HVPG of 10% or to ≤ 12 mmHg may be relevant in this setting. (1b;A)

Areas requiring further study
- Studies evaluating the use of carvedilol.
- Studies evaluating novel therapeutic options.

Lecture 10

Treatment of Acute Bleeding

Loren Laine[1], Shahab Abid[2], Agustin Albillos[3], Patrick S Kamath[4], Jean-Pierre Vinel[5] and Juan Carlos García-Pagán[6]

[1] Keck School of Medicine, University of Southern California, Los Angeles, CA, USA

[2] Department of Gastroenterology, Aga Khan University Hospital, Karachi, Pakistan

[3] Department of Gastroenterology, Hospital Ramon y Cajal, University of Alcalà, Madrid, Spain

[4] Mayo Clinic College of Medicine, Rochester, MN, USA

[5] Department of Hepato-Gastroenterology, University Hospital Toulouse-Purpan, and Inserm U858, Toulouse, France

[6] Hepatic Haemodynamic Laboratory, Liver Unit, Hospital Clinic, Institut d'Investigacions Biomèdiques August Pi i Sunyer (IDIBAPS) and Centro de Investigación Biomédica en Red de Enfermedades Hepáticas y Digestivas (CIBERehd), University of Barcelona, Spain

Introduction

Management of acute variceal bleeding (AVB) can be divided into three phases: *initial general management* includes resuscitation, airway protection, and prevention of potential complications such as infection; *primary therapy* of acute bleeding includes vasoactive medications and endoscopic treatment; *rescue therapy* is instituted in patients failing endoscopic-plus-medical management – usually with transjugular intrahepatic portosystemic shunt (TIPS).

General management
Resuscitation

The goal of early resuscitation in variceal bleeding is preservation of tissue oxygenation with correction of intravascular volume depletion and anaemia. Endotracheal intubation to protect the airway and prevent aspiration (e.g., with major ongoing bleeding, altered mental status) may be necessary.

Correcting hypovolaemia and anaemia

Fluid resuscitation must balance the risk of end-organ damage due to de-creased perfusion and the risk of perpetuating bleeding with overexpansion. Target systolic blood pressure of 90–100 mmHg and heart rate of 100 bpm with initial fluid resuscitation seem reasonable.

The target haemoglobin level is controversial. In experimental models of portal hypertension, total restitution of blood loss is associated with increased portal pressure and mortality [1,2]. A randomized trial in 214 cir-rhotics with gastrointestinal (GI) bleeding comparing a target haemoglobin of 7–8 g/dL vs. 9–10 g/dL [3] revealed significantly fewer therapeutic failures (16% vs. 28%) and non-significantly lower mortality (11% vs. 16%) with the restrictive strategy. Decisions in the individual patient should also consider factors such as age, comorbidities, haemodynamic status, and ongoing bleeding.

Correcting defects in haemostasis

Mild to moderate thrombocytopenia occurs in 50–65% of patients with advanced cirrhosis, but the platelet count is rarely lower than 30,000–40,000/mm^3 [4]. Thrombin generation in stable cirrhotic patients is similar to that of normal subjects with similar platelet counts [5]. Severe thrombocytopenia therefore might increase bleeding by reducing the number of thrombin-forming units, a rationale for platelet transfusion in cirrhotic patients with severe thrombocytopenia who are bleeding.

Cirrhotics have simultaneous impairment in the procoagulant factors (except for factor VIII and von Willebrand's) and anticoagulants (e.g. protein C, S) [6]. Conventional laboratory tests such as prothrombin time/INR, which measure procoagulant activity, are therefore unreliable in predicting coagulation status or bleeding risk and in guiding the use of plasma and other procoagulant factors. Plasma-based blood products are commonly used in cirrhotic patients with prolonged INR in spite of little supporting evidence of efficacy and known risks (volume expansion/overload, blood-borne infection, transfusion-related lung injury). Furthermore, the amount of plasma commonly employed is usually inadequate to correct the coagulopathy [7]. Indeed, 1 litre of plasma increases most clotting factors by only ∼10%. We lack controlled trials evaluating the efficacy and volume of fresh frozen plasma in prevention or treatment of bleeding in cirrhosis. Evidence from randomized controlled trials (RCTs) does not support the use of rFVIIa for variceal bleeding [8].

Prevention and management of complications
Bacterial infection

Bacterial infection complicated the course of 42% of cirrhotics after hospitalization with GI haemorrhage in a pooled analysis [9]. The most common infections are spontaneous bacterial peritonitis (SBP), bacteraemia, urinary tract infection, and pneumonia [10]. Meta-analysis of eight randomized trials comparing antibiotics to no therapy/placebo revealed a significant decrease in bacterial infections (18 vs. 42%; RR = 0.40, 95% Confidence intervals (C.I.) 0.32–0.51) and mortality (18 vs. 22%; RR = 0.73, 95% C.I. 0.55–0.95) [9]. Significant decreases were seen for bacteraemia, SBP, pneumonia, and urinary tract infection. Quinolones were the most commonly studied antibiotic, and results of the trials that used oral (4 trials) or intravenous followed by oral quinolones (three trials) were similar, leading the authors to suggest that oral quinolone therapy should be prescribed to eligible patients [9].

Gram-negative bacilli were previously the most frequent isolates. However, the spectrum of bacterial infection in patients with cirrhosis may have changed due to the extensive use of invasive procedures and long-term norfloxacin prophylaxis. In a prospective evaluation between 1998 and 2000, gram-positive cocci were responsible for 53% of bacterial infections in a liver unit and 37% of gram-negative isolates were quinolone-resistant [11].

For this reason, a randomized trial compared oral norfloxacin (400 mg bid) with intravenous ceftriaxone (1 g daily) for seven days in cirrhotics with GI bleeding and $\geq$ 2 of the following: ascites, severe malnutrition, encephalopathy, bilirubin > 3 g/dL [12]. Intravenous ceftriaxone was significantly more effective in preventing proven or possible infections (11% vs. 33%) and proven infections (11% vs. 26%), while in-hospital mortality was not significantly different (15% vs. 11%) [12]. The difference presumably related at least in part to lower efficacy of norfloxacin in a population with a high prevalence of norfloxacin-resistant bacteria. The results, however, may not be generalizable to cirrhotics as a whole because only 9% of screened patients were enrolled, with lack of advanced liver failure as the most common reason for exclusion. Intravenous ceftriaxone may be considered the option of choice in populations with severely decompensated cirrhosis, high prevalence of quinolone resistance, or prior quinolone prophylaxis.

Renal failure and ascites
Renal function should be supported by appropriate fluid resuscitation and avoiding drugs that worsen hypovolaemia (e.g. diuretics) or are nephrotoxic (e.g. NSAIDS, aminoglycosides). Tense ascites can contribute to dyspnoea and vomiting in patients with GI bleeding, and paracentesis can offer immediate relief. Large-volume paracentesis reduces portal pressure and portal-collateral blood flow [13], but can cause renal dysfunction in up to 18% of patients despite albumin replacement [14]. The alternative is smaller-volume (2–3 litres) paracentesis, which reduces intra-abdominal pressure and is associated with a low risk of renal dysfunction even without albumin [14].

Hepatic encephalopathy
GI haemorrhage often may precipitate hepatic encephalopathy. No RCTs document a significant benefit of therapy in preventing the development or treating an acute episode of hepatic encephalopathy in cirrhotics with GI bleeding.

Prognostic factors in acute variceal bleeding
Data on prognostic factors in AVB are largely derived from heterogeneous, often retrospective studies with variable definitions and out-of-date treatments, although several factors are consistent across multiple studies. HVPG > 20 mmHg, Child class C, and active bleeding are most consistently found to predict five-day treatment failure. These factors, together with systolic blood pressure < 100 mmHg and a non-alcoholic aetiology, independently predicted five-day treatment failure in the only study in which all patients received current standard treatment [15]. Other risk factors also identified in some studies are infections, high AST, active bleeding at endoscopy, blood transfusion, and portal vein thrombosis. Child class C, MELD score $\geq$ 18, and failure to control bleeding or early rebleeding consistently predict

six-week mortality; other factors are shock at admission, elevated HVPG, and hepatocellular carcinoma [16–23].

Conclusions regarding general management

Goals of initial management include airway protection and maintenance of tissue perfusion with cautious volume expansion to restore haemodynamic stability and a restricted packed red blood cell (PRBC) transfusion policy, targeting a haemoglobin of 7–8 g/dL. The prothrombin time/INR is not a reliable indicator of coagulation status or guide for use of fresh frozen plasma. Platelet transfusion may be considered in bleeding patients with severe thrombocytopenia but data documenting clinical benefit or transfusion thresholds are not available. Cirrhotic patients with upper GI bleeding should receive antibiotic prophylaxis. Oral quinolones are the first choice, but intravenous ceftriaxone is recommended with advanced cirrhosis and if risk of quinolone resistance is high.

Primary therapy for acute variceal bleeding
Balloon tamponade

Balloon tamponade is employed rarely and only in patients with massive bleeding as a temporary bridge (< 24 hours) until more definitive therapy can be provided [24]. A systematic review reported initial haemostasis in 90% of patients but permanent haemostasis in only 58%, with similar effectiveness for the Sengstaken-Blakemore (oesophageal and gastric balloons) and Linton-Nachlas (single large gastric balloon) tubes [25]. Complications occurred in 24% of patients (fatal in 5% of cases) and increased with duration of use [25].

Vasoactive medications

Vasoactive drugs are employed to decrease portal pressure and blood flow and thereby control variceal bleeding and prevent rebleeding. Vasopressin is no longer used due to side-effects such as ischaemia. Currently used medications include terlipressin or somatostatin and its analogues (e.g. octreotide, vapreotide). However, as discussed below, vasoactive drugs are used primarily in combination with endoscopic therapy.

Terlipressin

Four double-blind, placebo-controlled trials of terlipressin without endoscopic co-therapy revealed significantly better rates of bleeding control with terlipressin, with significant decreases in mortality in two trials [26–29]. Meta-analysis of five randomized trials of terlipressin vs. placebo/no active therapy revealed significant benefit both in failure to control bleeding (difference = 24%, 13–36%) and mortality (difference = 18%, 7–28%) [30].

Somatostatin and somatostatin analogues

Systematic review [31] reveals two published double-blind placebo-controlled trials assessing somatostatin without endoscopic co-therapy. One revealed significant benefit in failure of initial haemostasis (RR = 0.61, 0.41–0.90) and rebleeding (RR = 0.64, 0.45–0.91) [32], while the other showed no benefit: RR for failure of initial haemostasis = 2.13 (0.93–4.85) and rebleeding = 1.0 (0.24–4.19) [33]. One double-blind placebo-controlled trial assessing octreotide without endoscopic therapy showed no significant benefit: RR for failure of initial haemostasis = 0.96, 0.79–1.18 [34]. Vapreotide has not been assessed in a randomized trial without concomitant endoscopic therapy.

Dosing of vasoactive medications
Terlipressin is given at initial dose of 2 mg intravenously every four hours (1.5mg if 50–70kg and 1.0 mg if < 50kg) with titration to 1 mg every four hours considered after control of bleeding. Typically, somatostatin is administered as a 250 μg intravenous bolus followed by infusion of 250 μg/hour. Higher dose somatostatin (500 μg/hr) causes a greater fall in HVPG and may translate into better haemostatic efficacy and lower mortality in patients with active bleeding at endoscopy [35]. Octreotide and vapreotide are usually given as a 50 μg bolus followed by 50 μg/hour infusion.

Pre-endoscopic administration of vasoactive medications
Guidelines recommend initiation of vasoactive medications as soon as possible and prior to endoscopy in patients with suspected/potential variceal bleeding [24,36] on the basis of double-blind placebo-controlled trials that assessed vasoactive medications prior to endoscopy. Two trials showed significantly less active bleeding at initial endoscopy a mean of 3–4 hours after initiation of infusion (31% vs. 46% and 13% vs. 25%) [37,38] and the third showed significantly better bleeding control at 12 hours: 71% vs. 47% [29]. Unfortunately, these trials did not begin vasoactive drugs in the placebo group when varices were identified at endoscopy, so the benefit of pre-endoscopic therapy vs. initiation of vasoactive medications at endoscopy on post-endoscopic endpoints cannot be assessed.

Endoscopic treatment
Timing of endoscopy
Because ∼30% of patients with cirrhosis may have a non-variceal source of bleeding, endoscopy is essential to determine if varices are the cause of bleeding. Varices are considered the source of bleeding when blood is emanating from the varix, when stigmata of recent haemorrhage (e.g. white nipple sign, adherent clot) are seen, or if varices are noted with no other potential source. Early endoscopy within 24 hours after presentation is recommended in most patients who present with acute upper GI bleeding [39].

No randomized trials have studied the timing of endoscopy in cirrhotic patients with upper GI bleeding. A retrospective review of 210 patients hospitalized with haemodynamically stable variceal bleeding at presentation found that haemostasis rates were virtually identical when endoscopy was done ≤ or >12 hours. However, the 97% haemostasis rate indicates that all patients did exceptionally well initially and the study does not allow assessment of early endoscopy in a higher-risk population.

Previous guidelines suggest that any cirrhotic patient with upper GI bleeding should undergo endoscopy within 12 hours, regardless of the severity of bleeding [24,36] to obtain prognostic information (outcomes are worse with varices) and direct management. Furthermore, endoscopic therapy significantly improves outcomes in variceal bleeding, so earlier application may be beneficial.

Sclerotherapy

Endoscopic sclerotherapy controls active bleeding from varices in 62–100% of patients and is more effective than sham therapy or medical therapy with vasopressin or balloon tamponade in cessation of acute bleeding (OR = 8.5, C.I. 3.6–20.0), rebleeding during hospitalization or $\leq$ 2 wks (OR = 0.36, C.I. 0.21–0.62), and mortality (OR = 0.57, C.I. 0.33–0.98) [24].

Ligation

Two randomized trials specifically comparing ligation vs. sclerotherapy in AVB indicate ligation is significantly better in reducing further bleeding. Lo *et al.* [41] assessed 71 patients with active variceal bleeding and observed persistent bleeding of 3% with ligation vs. 24% with sclerotherapy at three days. Villanueva *et al.* [42] evaluated 179 patients with AVB and noted further bleeding of 4% with ligation vs. 15% with sclerotherapy at five days. Initial treatment of patients with actively bleeding varices occasionally may be more easily accomplished with sclerotherapy than ligation due to diminished visualization related to the friction-fit ligation cylinder.

Acute gastric variceal bleeding

For most type 2 gastro-oesophageal varices (GOV2), which are in continuity with oesophageal varices but extend into the fundus and tend to be longer and more tortuous, and for isolated gastric varices in the fundus (IGV1) and antrum (IGV2)), tissue adhesives are the current first-line treatment. N-butyl-2-cyanoacrylate is the agent most widely used around the world [43, 44]. In the USA, 2-octyl-cyanoacrylate, which has a longer polymerization time and is approved for cutaneous wound closure, is also used [45]. N-butyl-2-cyanoacrylate was significantly better than ligation in haemostasis within the subset of patients with actively bleeding gastric varices in one randomized trial (87% vs. 45%) [43] but not in a second randomized study (93% vs. 93%) [44]. In both trials, however, subsequent rebleeding was significantly lower with cyanoacrylate in the overall population. Gastro-oesophageal varices type 1 (GOV1) are an extension of oesophageal varices along the lesser curvature and may be managed with ligation or tissue adhesive. Case series also report control of bleeding gastric varices with thrombin or fibrin glue injection.

Endoscopic vs. medical therapy

A majority of available studies assessing endoscopic therapy against or in combination with medical therapy employed sclerotherapy. However, because ligation is more effective and has largely replaced sclerotherapy for treatment of oesophageal varices, these trials are not directly relevant to current practice.

A meta-analysis of RCTs comparing sclerotherapy to vasoactive drugs (primarily somatostatin or octreotide) for AVB revealed no significant differences in outcomes (difference in failure to control bleeding (14 studies) = –3% (C.I. –6 to 1%); difference in mortality (15 studies) = –4% (C.I. –7 to 1%)) but an increase in adverse events (difference in serious adverse events (3 studies) = 5% (C.I. 2 to 8%)) [46].

The one randomized trial comparing emergency ligation to vasoactive medication (somatostatin for 48 hours) in acute oesophageal variceal bleeding (N = 125) showed significantly better outcomes with ligation at 48 hours: treatment failure 5% vs. 30%; transfusions 4.7 vs. 6.9 units [47].

Combination endoscopic-medical therapy
Sclerotherapy plus vasoactive medications vs. vasoactive medications alone

In the one full manuscript assessing current vasoactive therapy (N = 100), sclerotherapy plus somatostatin for five days was significantly better than somatostatin alone for control of bleeding at both 24 hours (92% vs. 76%) and five days (86% vs. 58%) [48].

Ligation plus vasoactive medications vs. vasoactive medications alone

One randomized trial (N = 93) assessing ligation plus terlipressin for two days vs. terlipressin alone for five days showed that combination therapy was significantly better in preventing further bleeding at five days (2% vs. 24%) but not in failure to control bleeding within 48 hrs (2% vs. 9%) [49].

Sclerotherapy plus vasoactive medications vs. sclerotherapy alone

Several randomized trials show that a combination of somatostatin [37] or octreotide [50–53] plus sclerotherapy is significantly better than sclerotherapy alone at preventing further bleeding at five days and/or achieving initial haemostasis in ≤ 48 hours. A meta-analysis reported a significant benefit in control of bleeding with combined therapy (difference = 13.2%, C.I. 8.4–18.1%) without a significant difference in short-term (≤ six weeks) mortality (3.4%, C.I. –0.4 to 7.1%) [54].

Ligation plus vasoactive medications vs. ligation alone

A randomized trial (N = 94) showed that addition of octreotide for five days to ligation did not improve initial haemostasis vs. ligation alone (96% vs. 94%), but did significantly reduce further bleeding during hospitalization (13% vs. 45%); mortality was 9% vs. 19% (p = 0.135) [55]. Addition of somatostatin to ligation in another randomized trial (N = 47) was not significantly better than ligation alone (further bleeding within five days, 25% vs. 30%) [56].

TIPS or surgical shunt

Two randomized trials suggest that early use of TIPS in patients at high risk of treatment failure may be an appropriate initial treatment. One study randomized 52 patients with HVPG > 20 mmHg to uncoated TIPS within 24 hours (sclerotherapy was done at initial endoscopy in all patients) and reported significantly less failure to control acute bleeding (8% vs. 38%) and in-hospital mortality (11% vs. 38%) [22]. The second trial in 63 Child class C patients (with Child-Pugh score < 14) or class B patients with active variceal bleeding compared PTFE-coated TIPS within 72 hours to ligation/beta-blocker; all patients received endoscopic therapy and vasoactive drug at baseline [57]. Failure to control bleeding or prevent rebleeding (3% vs. 45%) and mortality (13% vs. 39%) were significantly better with TIPS at median follow-up of 16 months.

One surgical group reports excellent control of bleeding (100% at 14 days) and 10-year survival (46%) with emergency shunt surgery [58], although these results have not been replicated by others.

Conclusions regarding primary therapy

Vasoactive medications should be started as soon as possible and before endoscopy in patients with suspected/potential varices (e.g. cirrhotics). Endoscopy should be performed after initial resuscitation, within 12 hours of presentation. Ligation should be employed in patients with acute oesophageal variceal bleeding. If technical difficulty is encountered, sclerotherapy can be attempted instead. Co-therapy with vasoactive medications should be continued for up to five days. Although terlipressin shows the most robust results in placebo-controlled trials without endoscopic therapy, head-to-head studies of current vasoactive drugs, with and without endoscopic therapy, do not document superiority of any agent. TIPS may be appropriate primary therapy in selected high-risk patients (e.g. Child class C).

Rescue therapy for acute treatment failure

In 10–20% of patients variceal bleeding is unresponsive to initial endoscopic and/or pharmacologic treatment. If possible a second endoscopic therapy may be attempted, but if this fails or if the severity of bleeding precludes endoscopic therapy, another therapy should be employed. As discussed above, balloon tamponade occasionally may be attempted, but only for a short time in cases of massive bleeding as a temporary bridge to definitive treatment.

Self-expanding metal stent

Placement of a covered self-expanding metal stent has recently been reported [59,60]. In the largest series, 34 patients whose acute oesophageal variceal bleeding "could not be managed using standard therapy" had stents of the authors' design placed, with cessation of bleeding in all and no rebleeding [59]. Stent migration occurred in seven patients, but the stent was repositioned endoscopically 1–2 days later. The stent was removed at a mean of five days (range, 1–14 days) and the only complication was an oesophageal ulcer in one patient. Further assessment is required to determine the role of stenting in oesophageal variceal bleeding.

Transjugular intrahepatic portosystemic shunts (TIPS) or surgical shunts

TIPS and surgical shunts are extremely effective in controlling variceal bleeding (approaching 95%), but due to worsening of liver function and encephalopathy, mortality remains high. TIPS is generally the first choice for salvage therapy because most patients requiring rescue treatment have advanced liver disease with high surgical risk. TIPS with uncoated stents has similar efficacy to surgical shunt in well-compensated cirrhotics with refractory variceal bleeding, but requires significantly more reinterventions [61]. However, PTFE-coated stents have reduced shunt dysfunction, clinical relapse, and need for re-intervention and are the stents of choice for TIPS [62].

Conclusions regarding rescue therapy

TIPS with PTFE-coated stent is the treatment of choice in most patients who fail medical and endoscopic therapy. Initial reports of self-expanding oesophageal metal stents are promising but further evaluation is needed.

References

1. Castañeda B, Debernardi-Venon W, Bandi JC, *et al.* (2000) The role of portal pressure in the severity of bleeding in portal hypertensive rats. *Hepatology* **31**:581–6.
2. Kravetz D, Sikuler E, Groszmann RJ (1986) Splanchnic and systemic hemodynamics in portal hypertensive rats during hemorrhage and blood volume restitution. *Gastroenterology* **90**:1232–40.
3. Colomo A, Hernández-Gea V, Muñiz-Díaz E, *et al.* (2008) Transfusion strategies in patients with cirrhosis and acute gastrointestinal bleeding. *Hepatology* **48**:413A.
4. Bashour FN, Teran JC, Mullen KD, *et al.* (2000) Prevalence of peripheral blood cytopenias (hypersplenism) in patients with nonalcoholic chronic liver disease. *Am J Gastroenterol* **95**:2936–9.
5. Tripodi A, Primignani M, Chantarangkul V, *et al.* (2006) Thrombin generation in patients with cirrhosis: the role of platelets. *Hepatology* **44**:440–5.
6. Tripodi A, Primignani M, Chantarangkul V, *et al.* (2009) An imbalance of pro- vs. anti-coagulation factors in plasma from patients with cirrhosis. *Gastroenterology* **137**:2105–11.
7. Youssef WI, Salazar F, Dasarathy S, Beddow T, Mullen KD. (2003) Role of fresh frozen plasma infusion in correction of coagulopathy of chronic liver disease: a dual phase study. *Am J Gastroenterol* **98**:1391–4.
8. Bosch J, Thabut D, Albillos A, *et al.* (2008) Recombinant factor VIIa for variceal bleeding in patients with advanced cirrhosis: A randomized, controlled trial. *Hepatology* **47**:1604–14.
9. Soares-Weiser K, Brezis M, Tur-Kaspa R, Leibovici L (2002) Antibiotic prophylaxis for cirrhotic patients with gastrointestinal bleeding. *Cochrane Database Syst Rev*, CD002907.

10. Garcia-Tsao G (2004) Treatment of acute variceal bleeding: general management and prevention of infections. In: Groszmann RJ, Bosch J (eds) *Portal Hypertension in the 21st Century.* Kluwer Academic Publishers: Dordrecht, pp. 233–40.

11. Fernández J, Navasa M, Gómez J, *et al.* (2002) Bacterial infections in cirrhosis: epidemiological changes with invasive procedures and norfloxacin prophylaxis. *Hepatology* **35**:140–8.

12. Fernández J, Ruiz-del-Arbol L, Gómez C, *et al.* (2006) Norfloxacin vs. ceftriaxone in the prophylaxis of infections in patients with advanced cirrhosis and hemorrhage. *Gastroenterology* **131**:1049–56.

13. Luca A, Feu F, García-Pagán JC, *et al.* (1994) Favorable effects of total paracentesis on splanchnic haemodynamics in cirrhotic patients with tense ascites. *Hepatology* **20**:30–3.

14. Ginès A, Fernández-Esparrach G, Monescillo A, *et al.* (1996) Randomized trial comparing albumin, dextran 70, and polygeline in cirrhotic patients with ascites treated by paracentesis. *Gastroenterology* **111**:1002–10.

15. Abraldes JG, Villanueva C, Bañares R, *et al.* (2008) Hepatic venous pressure gradient and prognosis in patients with acute variceal bleeding treated with pharmacologic and endoscopic therapy. *J Hepatol* **48**:229–36.

16. Gatta A, Merkel C, Amodio P, *et al.* (1994) Development and validation of a prognostic index predicting death after upper gastrointestinal bleeding in patients with liver cirrhosis: a multicenter study. *Am J Gastroenterol* **89**:1528–36.

17. Ben Ari Z, Cardin F, McCormick AP, Wannamethee G, Burroughs AK (1999) A predictive model for failure to control bleeding during acute variceal haemorrhage. *J Hepatol* **31**:443–50.

18. Moitinho E, Escorsell A, Bandi JC, *et al.* (1999) Prognostic value of early measurements of portal pressure in acute variceal bleeding. *Gastroenterology* **117**:626–31.

19. D'Amico G, de Franchis R (2003) Upper digestive bleeding in cirrhosis. Posttherapeutic outcome and prognostic indicators. *Hepatology* **38**:599–612.

20. Villanueva C, Ortiz J, Minana J, *et al.* (2001) Somatostatin treatment and risk stratification by continuous portal pressure monitoring during acute variceal bleeding. *Gastroenterology* **121**:110–17.

21. Cardenas A, Gines P, Uriz J, *et al.* (2001) Renal failure after upper gastrointestinal bleeding in cirrhosis: incidence, clinical course, predictive factors, and short-term prognosis. *Hepatology* **34**:671–6.

22. Monescillo A, Martinez-Lagares F, Ruiz-del-Arbol L, *et al.* (2004) Influence of portal hypertension and its early decompression by TIPS placement on the outcome of variceal bleeding. *Hepatology* **40**:793–801.

23. Avgerinos A, Armonis A, Stefanidis G, *et al.* (2004) Sustained rise of portal pressure after sclerotherapy, but not band ligation, in acute variceal bleeding in cirrhosis. *Hepatology* **39**:1623–30.

24. Laine L, Planas R, Nevens F, *et al.* (2006) Treatment of the acute bleeding episode. In: de Franchis R (ed.) *Portal Hypertension IV. Proceedings of the Fourth Baveno International Consensus Workshop on Methodology of Diagnosis and Treatment.* Blackwell Publishing: Oxford, pp. 217–42.

25. Avgerinos A, Armonis A (1994) Balloon tamponade technique and efficacy in variceal haemorrhage. *Scand J Gastroenterol* **29** (Suppl 207): 11–16.

26. Walker S, Stiehl A, Raedsch R, Kommerell B (1986) Terlipressin in bleeding esophageal varices: a placebo-controlled, double-blind study. *Hepatology* **6**:112–15.

27. Freeman JG, Cobden I, Record CO (1989) Placebo-controlled trial of ter-lipressin (glypressin) in the management of acute variceal bleeding. *J Clin Gastroenterol* **11**:58–60.

28. Soderlund C, Magnusson I, Torngren S, Lundell L (1990) Terlipressin (triglycyl-lysine vasopressin) controls acute bleeding oesophageal varices. A double-blind, randomized, placebo-controlled trial. *Scand J Gastroenterol* **25**:622–30.

29. Levacher S, Letoumelin P, Pateron D, *et al.* (1995) Early administration of terli-pressin plus glyceryl trinitrate to control active upper gastrointestinal bleeding in cirrhotic patients. *Lancet* **346**:865–8.

30. D'Amico G, Pagliaro L, Bosch J (1999) Pharmacological treatment of portal hypertension: an evidence-based approach. *Sem Liv Dis* **19**:475–505.

31. Gøtzsche PC, Hróbjartsson A (2008) Somatostatin analogues for acute bleed-ing oesophageal varices. *Cochrane Database Syst Rev* (3): CD000193. DOI: 10.1002/14651858.CD000193.pub3.

32. Burroughs AK, McCormick PA, Hughes MD, *et al.* (1990) Randomized, double-blind, placebo controlled trial of somatostatin for variceal bleed-ing. Emergency control and prevention of early rebleeding. *Gastroenterology* **99**:1388–95.

33. Valenzuela JE, Schubert T, Fogel MR, *et al.* (1989) A multicenter, randomized, double-blind trial of somatostatin in the management of acute hemorrhage from esophageal varices. *Hepatology* **10**:958–61.

34. Burroughs AK (1996) Double blind RCT of 5 day octreotide versus placebo, associated with sclerotherapy for trial/failures. *Hepatology* **24**:352A.

35. Moitinho E, Planas R, Bañares R, *et al.*, Variceal Bleeding Study Group (2001) Multicenter randomized controlled trial comparing different sched-ules of somatostatin in the treatment of acute variceal bleeding. *J Hepatol* **35**: 712–18.

36. Garcia-Tsao G, Sanyal AJ, Grace ND, Carey WD (2007) Prevention and man-agement of gastroesophageal varices and variceal hemorrhage in cirrhosis. *Am J Gastroenterol* **102**:2086–102.

37. Avgerinos A, Nevens F, Raptis S, Fevery J (1997) Early administration of so-matostatin and efficacy of sclerotherapy in acute oesophageal variceal bleeds: the European Acute Bleeding Oesophageal Variceal Episodes (ABOVE) ran-domised trial. *Lancet* **350**:1495–9.

38. Calès P, Masliah C, Bernard B, *et al.* (2001) Early administration of vapreotide for variceal bleeding in patients with cirrhosis. *N Engl J Med* **344**:23–8.

39. Barkun A, Bardou M, Kuipers C, *et al.* (2010) International consensus recom-mendations on the management of patients with non-variceal upper gastroin-testinal bleeding. *Ann Intern Med* **152**:101–13.

40. Cheung J, Soo I, Bastiampillai R, Zhu Q, Ma M (2009) Urgent vs. non-urgent endoscopy in stable acute variceal bleeding. *Am J Gastroenterol* **104**:1125–9.

41. Lo GH, Lai KH, Cheng JS, *et al.* (1997) Emergency banding ligation ver-sus sclerotherapy for the control of active bleeding from esophageal varices. *Hepatology* **25**:1101–4.

42. Villanueva C, Piqueras M, Aracil C, et al. (2006) A randomized controlled trial comparing ligation and sclerotherapy as emergency endoscopic treatment added to somatostatin in acute variceal bleeding. *J Hepatol* **45**:560–7.

43. Lo GH, Lai KH, Cheng JS, Chen MH, Chiang HT (2001) A prospective, randomized trial of butyl cyanoacrylate injection versus band ligation in the management of bleeding gastric varices. *Hepatology* **33**:1060–4.

44. Tan PC, Hou MC, Lin HC, *et al.* (2006) A randomized trial of endoscopic treatment of acute gastric variceal hemorrhage: N-butyl-2-cyanoacrylate injection versus band ligation. *Hepatology* **43**:690–7.

45. Rengstorff DS, Binmoeller KF (2004) A pilot study of 2-octyl cyanoacrylate injection for treatment of gastric fundal varices in humans. *Gastrointest Endosc* **59**:553–8.

46. D'Amico G, Pietrosi G, Tarantino I, Pagliaro L (2003) Emergency sclerotherapy versus vasoactive drugs for variceal bleeding in cirrhosis: A Cochrane meta-analysis. *Gastroenterology* **124**:1277–91.

47. Chen WC, Lo GH, Tsai WL, *et al.* (2006) Emergency endoscopic variceal ligation versus somatostatin for acute esophageal variceal bleeding. *J Chinese Med Assoc* **69**:55–7.

48. Villaneueva C, Ortiz J, Sabat M, *et al.* (1999) Somatostatin alone or combined with emergency sclerotherapy in the treatment of acute esophageal variceal bleeding: a prospective randomized trial. *Hepatology* **30**:384–9.

49. Lo GH, Chen WC, Wang HM, *et al.* (2009) Low-dose terlipressin plus banding ligation versus low-dose terlipressin alone in the prevention of very early rebleeding of oesophageal varices. *Gut* **58**:1275–80.

50. Besson I, Ingrand P, Person B, *et al.* (1995) Sclerotherapy with or without octreotide for acute variceal bleeding. *N Engl J Med* **333**:555–60.

51. Zuberi BF, Baloch Q (2000) Comparison of endoscopic variceal sclerotherapy alone and in combination with octreotide in controlling acute variceal hemorrhage and early rebleeding in patients with low-risk cirrhosis. *Am J Gastroenterol* **95**:768–71.

52. Freitas SD, Sofia C, Pontes JM, *et al.* (2000) Octreotide in acute bleeding esophageal varices: a prospective randomized study. *Hepatogastroenterology* **47**:1310–14.

53. Shah HA, Mumtaz K, Jafri W, *et al.* (2005) Sclerotherapy plus octreotide versus sclerotherapy alone in the management of gastro-oesophageal variceal hemorrhage. *J Ayub Med Coll Abbottabad* **17**:10–14.

54. Triantos CK, Patch D, Papatheodordis GV, *et al.* (2006) An evaluation of emergency sclerotherapy of varices in randomized trials: looking the needle in the eye. *Endoscopy* **38**:E74–90.

55. Sung JJY, Chung SCS, Yung MY, *et al.* (1995) Prospective randomised study of effect of octreotide on rebleeding from oesophageal varices after endoscopic ligation. *Lancet* **346**:1666–9.

56. Sarin SK, Kumar A, Jha SK, Sharma P, Sharma B (2008) Combination of somatostatin plus endoscopic variceal ligation (EVL) is similar to EVL alone in control of acute variceal bleeding: a randomized controlled trial. *Hepatology* **48** (Suppl): 628A.

57. García-Pagán JC, Caca K, Bureau C, *et al.* (2010) Early use of TIPS in patients with cirrhosis and variceal bleeding. *N Engl J Med* **362**:2370–9.

58. Orloff MJ, Isenberg JI, Wheeler HO, *et al.* (2009) Randomized trial of emergency endoscopic sclerotherapy versus emergency portacaval shunt for acutely bleeding esophageal varices in cirrhosis. *J Am Coll Surg* **209**: 25–40.

59. Zehetner J, Shamiyeh A, Wayand W, Hubmann R (2008) Results of a new method to stop acute bleeding from esophageal varices: implantation of a self-expanding stent. *Surg Endosc* **22**:2149–52.

60. Wright G, Lewis H, Hogan B, *et al.* (2010) A self-expanding metal stent for complicated variceal hemorrhage: experience at a single center. *Gastrointest Endosc* **71**:71–8.

61. Henderson JM, Boyer TD, Kutner MH, *et al.* (2006) Distal splenorenal shunt versus transjugular intrahepatic portal systematic shunt for variceal bleeding: a randomized trial. *Gastroenterology* **130**:1643–51.

62. Bureau C, García-Pagán JC, Layrargues GP, *et al.* (2007) Patency of stents covered with polytetrafluoroethylene in patients treated by transjugular intrahepatic portosystemic shunts: long-term results of a randomized multicentre study. *Liver Int* **27**:742–74.

Treatment of the Acute Bleeding Episode

Juan Carlos García-Pagán, Loren Laine (Chairpersons), Shahab Abid, Agustin Albillos, Patrick Kamath and Jean-Pierre Vinel

Blood volume restitution

- The goal of resuscitation is to preserve tissue perfusion. Volume restitution should be initiated to restore and maintain haemodynamic stability.
- PRBC transfusion should be done conservatively at a target haemoglobin level between 7–8 g/dL, although transfusion policy in individual patients should also consider other factors such as co-morbidities, age, haemodynamic status and ongoing bleeding. (1;A)
- Recommendations regarding management of coagulopathy and thrombocytopenia cannot be made on the basis of currently available data.
- PT/INR is not a reliable indicator of the coagulation status in patients with cirrhosis.

Antibiotic prophylaxis

- Antibiotic prophylaxis is an integral part of therapy for patients with cirrhosis presenting with upper gastrointestinal bleeding and should be instituted from admission. (1;A)
- Oral quinolones are recommended for most patients. (1;A)
- Intravenous ceftriaxone should be considered in patients with advanced cirrhosis (1;A), in hospital settings with high prevalence of quinolone-resistant bacterial infections and in patients on previous quinolone prophylaxis. (1;C)

Prevention of hepatic encephalopathy

- Recommendations regarding management and prevention of encephalopathy in patients with cirrhosis and upper GI bleeding cannot be made on the basis of currently available data. (5;D)

Assessment of prognosis

- HVPG ≥ 20 mmHg, Child class C, and active bleeding at endoscopy are the variables most consistently found to predict five-day treatment failure. (2b;B)

Portal Hypertension V, 5th edition. Edited by Roberto de Franchis.
© 2011 Blackwell Publishing Ltd.

- Child class C, MELD score ≥18, and failure to control bleeding or early rebleeding are the variables most consistently found to predict six-week mortality. (2b;B)

Timing of endoscopy

- Patients with GI bleeding and features suggesting cirrhosis should have upper endoscopy as soon as possible after admission (within 12 hours). (5;D)

Pharmacological treatment

- In suspected variceal bleeding, vasoactive drugs should be started as soon as possible, before endoscopy. (1b;A)
- Vasoactive drugs (terlipressin, somatostatin, octreotide, vapreotide) should be used in combination with endoscopic therapy and continued for up to five days. (1a;A)

Endoscopic treatment

- Endoscopic therapy is recommended in any patient who presents with documented upper GI bleeding and in whom oesophageal varices are the cause of bleeding. (1a;A)
- Ligation is the recommended form of endoscopic therapy for acute oesophageal variceal bleeding, although sclerotherapy may be used in the acute setting if ligation is technically difficult. (1b;A)
- Endoscopic therapy with tissue adhesive (e.g. N-butyl-cyanoacrylate) is recommended for acute bleeding from isolated gastric varices (IGV) (1b;A) and those gastro-oesophageal varices type 2 (GOV2) that extend beyond the cardia. (5;D)
- EVL or tissue adhesive can be used in bleeding from gastro-oesophageal varices type 1 (GOV1). (5;D)

Early TIPS placement

- An early TIPS within 72 hours (ideally ≤ 24 hours) should be considered in patients at high risk of treatment failure (e.g. Child class C < 14 points or Child class B with active bleeding) after initial pharmacological and endoscopic therapy. (1b;A)

Use of balloon tamponade

- Balloon tamponade should only be used in massive bleeding as a temporary "bridge" until definitive treatment can be instituted (for a maximum of 24 hours, preferably in an intensive care facility). (5;D)

Use of self-expandable metal stents

- Uncontrolled data suggest that self-expanding covered oesophageal metal stent may be an option in refractory oesophageal variceal bleeding, although further evaluation is needed. (4;C)

Management of treatment failures

- Persistent bleeding despite combined pharmacological and endoscopic therapy is best managed by TIPS with PTFE-covered stents. (2b;B)
- Rebleeding during the first five days may be managed by a second attempt at endoscopic therapy. If rebleeding is severe, PTFE-covered TIPS is likely the best option. (2b;B)

Areas requiring further study

- The need for correction of coagulation disorders. Influence of coagulopathy and thrombocytopenia on outcome.
- Improve prognostic models: better stratification of risk to determine timing of the initial endoscopy, duration of drug therapy and type of treatment.
- Treatment and prevention of HE.
- Best antibiotic.
- Role of self-expandable oesophageal stents.
- Treatment of gastric varices.
- Treatment of paediatric patients: no studies define the best approach.
- Treatment of bleeding ectopic varices like duodenal varices.
- Role of erythromycin before endoscopy.

Lecture 11
Preventing Rebleeding in 2010

**Norman Grace[1], Gin-Ho Lo[2], Frederik Nevens[3],
Tilman Sauerbruch[4], Peter Hayes[5], Candid Villanueva[6] and
Didier Lebrec[7]**

[1]Department of Medicine, Tufts University School of Medicine; Harvard Medical School, and
Department of Clinical Hepatology, Brigham and Women's Hospital, Boston, MA, USA
[2]Department of Medical Nutrition, I-Shou University, and Digestive Centre, E-DA Hospital,
Kaohsiung, Taiwan
[3]Department of Liver and Pancreatic Disease, UZ Gasthuisberg KU Leuven, Leuven, Belgium
[4]Department of Internal Medicine I, University of Bonn, Germany
[5]Department of Hepatology, University of Edinburgh, UK
[6]Department of Gastroenterology, Hospital de la Santa Creu i Sant Pau, Barcelona, Spain
[7]Inserm U773, Centre de Recherche Biomédicale Bichat-Beaujon CRB3, Université Denis Diderot
Paris 7, and Department of Hepatology, Hôpital Beaujon, Clichy, France

Beta-blockers alone or combined with other drugs

Previous Baveno consensus conferences have concluded that non-selective
beta-blockers (NSBBs) are effective in decreasing the risk of recurrent
variceal haemorrhage and mortality [1]. Meta-analyses show a reduction
in rebleeding from 63% for patients treated with placebo or no treatment to
42% for patients receiving NSBBs. Mortality is similarly reduced from 27%
to 20%. The NNT for prevention of rebleeding is 5 and for prevention of
mortality, 14.

Vasodilators such as isosorbide-5-mononitrate (ISMN) increase the number of haemodynamic responders. Studies comparing the combination of a
beta-blocker and ISMN to beta-blocker monotherapy have been inconclu-
sive in showing a benefit either for prevention of rebleeding or for survival.
However, limited human studies have shown variable results and side-effects
such as systemic hypotension may limit their use.

In summary, beta-blocker monotherapy is very effective for the minority
of patients achieving a significant haemodynamic response to treatment. The
remaining majority will require combination therapy using a beta-blocker
combined with additional agents and/or procedures.

Endoscopic therapy: endoscopic variceal ligation or combined with other endoscopic procedures

Endoscopic injection sclerotherapy (EIS) took a leading role in 1980s in the
prevention of variceal rebleeding, but is now almost completely replaced by
endoscopic variceal ligation (EVL), owing to higher complication rates and
lower effectiveness in the reduction of rebleeding episodes [2]. Because of

Portal Hypertension V, 5th edition. Edited by Roberto de Franchis.
© 2011 Blackwell Publishing Ltd.

the different action mechanisms of EIS and EVL, combining EIS and EVL to hasten eradication of varices was attempted. The combination of EIS and EVL can be synchronous or metachronous. A meta-analysis of synchronous combination studies showed that combination therapy may lengthen the treatment time and is associated with a higher rate of oesophageal strictures. Hou *et al.* tried to bind varices initially, then perform sclerotherapy, and finally ligation once again, (so-called "sandwich" method) during the same treatment session [3]. The results showed that combination could further reduce variceal rebleeding as compared with treatment with EVL alone. Synchronous combination of EVL and endoscopic injection sclerotherapy has been generally discarded. On the other hand, several trials have shown that metachronous combination therapy of EIS and EVL could reduce the variceal recurrence or even reduce incidence of variceal rebleeding as compared with treatment with EVL or endoscopic injection sclerotherapy alone.

To reduce variceal recurrence, the addition of microwave in patients receiving repeated EVL was shown to be comparable to sclerotherapy. Nakamura and colleagues adopted argon plasma coagulation (APC) following variceal obliteration achieved by EVL. The study demonstrated that variceal recurrence decreased from 74% in patients receiving EVL alone to 49 % in patients receiving argon plasma as a "consolidation therapy" of repeated EVL [4]. A similar study from Italy showed that variceal recurrence could decrease from 42% in patients treated with EVL alone to 0% in patients treated with APC following repeated EVL. It appears that the addition of either sclerotherapy, microwave or argon plasma following variceal obliteration achieved by EVL could effectively reduce variceal recurrence. Combinations of EVL and microwave or argon plasma require further controlled studies before they can be universally recommended.

Drugs alone or with endoscopic variceal ligation? Endoscopic variceal ligation alone or with drugs?

An aggressive approach is justified in case of secondary prophylaxis. Since NSBBs protect against rebleeding before the varices are obliterated by endotherapy and since they delay recurrence of varices, the combination of endoscopic therapy together with drugs is the most rational strategy to prevent variceal rebleeding. This is supported by a meta-analysis [5]. A difference in survival has never been observed in any of the studies that investigated secondary prophylaxis of variceal bleeding.

Endoscopic variceal ligation and drugs vs. ligation alone

Two randomized trials confirmed the superiority of the combination of EVL and drugs versus EVL alone (Table 1) [7, 8]. In a third study the addition of beta-blockers plus ISMN to EVL did not reduce the incidence of variceal rebleeding but increased the occurrence of severe adverse events.

Endoscopic variceal ligation vs. combination of drugs

If one focuses on the four trials that compared EVL vs. drug combination there was no difference in rebleeding rate (Table 2). A recent meta-analysis of these trials showed a higher rebleeding rate on beta-blockers if the mean

Table 1

First author (ref)		Overall rebleeding	Variceal rebleeding	Adverse events	Follow-up (month)
Lo [6]	EVL (n = 62) vs. EVL+nadolol (n = 60)	47 vs. 23% p = 0.005	29 vs. 12% p = 0.01	8 vs. 12%	21
de la Peña [7]	EVL (n = 37) vs. EVL+nadolol (n = 43)	38 vs. 14% p = 0.006	27 vs. 9%	3 vs. 33%	16

daily dosage was less than 80 mg [12]. Moreover in the only study which was in favour of EVL, long-term follow-up showed higher overall and higher liver-related mortality despite a lower rebleeding rate.

Combination of drugs vs. endoscopic variceal ligation and combination of drugs

Whether EVL is indeed necessary has been questioned recently by the long-term outcome of the study by Lo *et al.* and by two recent studies that demonstrated that patients treated by EVL had indeed less spontaneous bleeding from varices but this beneficial effect was counteracted by an increased risk of EVL-induced bleeding (Table 3).

Conclusions

A combination of EVL and NSBBs can be considered as the treatment of choice in the prevention of variceal rebleeding. There are not enough data to support the need to add ISMN to beta-blockers in this condition.

Table 2

First author [ref]		Overall rebleeding	Variceal rebleeding	Adverse events	Follow-up (months)
Villanueva [8]	EVL (n=72) vs. nadolol + ISMN (n = 72)	49 vs. 33% p = 0.04	44 vs. 28% p = 0.04	12 vs. 3% p = 0.05	21
Lo [9]	EVL (n = 60) vs. nadolol + ISMN (n = 61)	38 vs. 57 % p = 0.10	20 vs. 42% p = 0.01	17 vs. 19%	25
Patch [10]	EVL (n = 51) vs. propranolol + ISMN (n = 51)	53 vs. 37%	35 vs. 22%	14 vs. 20%	10
Romero [11]	EVL (n = 52) vs. nadolol + ISMN (n = 57)	46 vs. 47%	33 vs. 37%	14 vs. 7%	18

Table 3

First author [ref]		Overall rebleeding	Variceal rebleeding	Adverse events	Follow-up (months)
García-Pagán [13]	nadolol+ISMN (n =78) vs. EVL+drugs (n = 80)	35 vs. 28%	32 vs. 18% p = 0.03	32 vs. 61% p < 0.01	15
Lo [14]	nadolol+ISMN (n = 60) vs. EVL+drugs (n = 60)	51 vs. 38%	43 vs. 26% p = 0.07	60 vs. 50%	23

Transjugular intrahepatic portosystemic shunt versus endoscopic treatment

Twelve randomized controlled trials were performed comparing TIPS to endoscopic treatment for secondary prophylaxis [15]. These studies are variable in terms of number of subjects with advanced liver failure, nature of endoscopic treatment used (sclerotherapy vs. band ligation), use of pharmacologic agents along with endoscopic treatment, timing of TIPS with respect to the initial presentation with bleeding and sample size. Most studies did not provide the data normally captured in a CONSORT diagram. Importantly, virtually all trials were performed before the availability of covered stents and thus utilized bare stents.

These trials included a total of 883 subjects. A total of 280 subjects rebled (86 treated with TIPS versus 194 with endoscopic treatment). In a fixed effects model, TIPS was found to have a pooled odds ratio 0.32 (0.24–0.43, 95% C.I., p < 0.00001) indicating that it was substantially superior to endoscopy with respect to prevention of variceal rebleeding [15]. However, this did not translate into a survival advantage for subjects undergoing TIPS. It has recently been further observed that, although overall mortality did not decrease, rebleeding-related deaths were significantly decreased in those who received a TIPS (odds ratio: 0.35, p < 0.002) [15]. TIPS was also associated with a significantly greater risk of developing encephalopathy; however, only a few subjects developed severe refractory encephalopathy. The use of covered stents has significantly reduced the need for repeated interventions after TIPS.

An important study measured HVPG within 12–24 hours after initial control of bleeding and randomized subjects with a HVPG ≥20 mmHg to endoscopic treatment vs. TIPS. TIPS was associated with improvement both in rebleeding and survival. These data have been corroborated in another trial recently published [16]. A small recent trial found a lower rebleeding rate with TIPS compared to cyanoacrylate injection for gastric variceal haemorrhage. However, the rebleeding rates with cyanoacrylate were higher than those reported in the literature.

Rescue therapy: always TIPS? Treatment of poor candidates for TIPS

In unselected and selected patients it has been shown that immediate place-ment of an open surgical shunt or a TIPS [17] is the most effective method to treat bleeding and to prevent rebleeding. This may improve survival. Pa-tients with a high portal pressure (HVPG > 20 mmHg) may benefit from TIPS placement. Most Child A/B patients with active variceal bleeding or signs of very recent bleeding have a HVPG > 20 mmHg.

Although shunts are effective, there are patients unfit for TIPS, and it is unclear how to treat these patients.

Definition

1. Failure to control bleeding has been defined in Baveno IV.
2. Very early rebleeding is defined as an event occurring between day 2 and day 5 after onset of treatment, and
3. Early rebleeding as rebleeding within day 42 after the initial event.
   We suggest applying the term *rescue therapy* to one of the above situations.

Available methods

(a) TIPS directed by haemodynamic monitoring or clinical/laboratory pa-rameters
(b) endoscopy (ligation, injection)
(c) balloon tamponade
(d) stents.

Results

Uncontrolled trials show that for the situation 1 and 2 of the definition TIPS has a high risk of a 30-day mortality of around 30–40%. In selected high-risk patients immediate TIPS has a considerably lower mortality. How-ever, patients with a Child-Pugh grade greater than 13 were excluded. It is unknown whether immediate shunt is beneficial also in these extremely sick patients.

Balloon tamponade in situation 1 and 2 achieves haemostasis in up to 60–90% of patients for a short time with a rebleeding rate of 50% and a rather high complication rate.

On the whole, endoscopic haemostasis is inferior to TIPS. However, en-doscopic injection of glue is commonly used in the treatment of gastric varices. Here, it is superior to band ligation. It is unclear whether injection of glue in oesophageal varices is an effective rescue therapy.

Some small uncontrolled series suggest that self-expanding metal stents may be used to compress the bleeding varices with a haemostasis rate of 90–100% without major complications. These stents are intended as bridg-ing procedures until more definitive procedures such as shunts or liver transplantation can be implemented. Rescue therapy for early rebleeding (No. 3 definition) depends on the therapy for primary bleeding and degree of liver dysfunction.

Prognosis

Several prognostic scores have been evaluated. An APACHE score higher than 17, a MELD score higher than 20, or a Child-Pugh score higher than 11 are accompanied with a 30-day mortality between 40–60%, no matter which therapy is used to treat/prevent bleeding. Bilirubin and kidney function are important independent prognostic variables. The sicker the patient the more important it is to achieve definitive haemostasis.

Secondary prophylaxis of variceal bleeding: Role of surgery

With the development of pharmacological, endoscopic and radiological treatment of portal hypertension and variceal haemorrhage the role of surgery to prevent variceal rebleeding has decreased over the last three decades.

Surgery for variceal bleeding can be divided into portosystemic shunt surgery, oesophageal transection and liver transplantation. Transplantation would rarely be considered for secondary prophylaxis of variceal bleeding and oesophageal transection or devascularization surgery is now infrequently undertaken to control acute bleeding. Some data regarding portosystemic shunt surgery in comparison to alternative treatments exist and are reasonably consistent.

Three papers of total surgical shunt surgery vs. endoscopic therapy show a significant reduction in rebleeding (OR 0.14) but with more encephalopathy (OR 1.52) and similar mortality (OR 1.03). Four studies of distal splenorenal shunt (DSRS) surgery vs. endoscopic therapy report similar findings to total surgical shunt surgery although chronic encephalopathy was not different (OR 1.29) [18]. In the era of liver transplantation portocaval shunts are avoided in potential candidates. It should be remembered also that the endoscopic therapy used in these trials was sclerotherapy rather than band ligation.

DSRS and TIPS have recently been compared for prevention of rebleeding in patients with refractory variceal bleeding and were shown to be equally effective. Reintervention was more common for TIPS, but uncovered stents were used [19]. The authors' conclusion was that the choice was dependent upon available expertise. TIPS may not be possible in patients with cirrhosis and complications such as portal vein thrombosis, or in patients with extrahepatic portal hypertension, and in this setting portosystemic shunt surgery may be valuable [20].

In conclusion, surgery is seldom required in the secondary prophylaxis of variceal haemorrhage but may be considered in selected cases such as those with portal vein thrombosis. Expertise and experience with the surgical techniques is decreasing.

The role of HVPG monitoring in secondary prophylaxis

HVPG monitoring is a valid surrogate endpoint to predict clinical outcomes in cirrhosis with portal hypertension that may be particularly useful in the high-risk setting of preventing rebleeding [21]. HVPG monitoring provides strong prognostic information adequately identifying haemodynamic responders, (with a decrease in HVPG to <12 mmHg or by > 20% from baseline), who have a marked reduction of rebleeding risk to below 15%. With such a low risk, comparable to that achieved with portal-systemic shunts, it is unlikely that responders will need further therapy. Even when response occurs spontaneously, in patients treated only with EVL, it is associated with lower probability of rebleeding and better survival [9].

Some issues should be considered to improve HVPG monitoring, particularly in secondary prophylaxis. Control measurement should be performed in less than one month after the baseline, because rebleeding can occur within this time frame. Furthermore, given that about half non-responders do not bleed, prognostic indicators are needed to identify non-responders at real risk. Moreover, recent studies have shown that acute response to beta-blockers in a single study may provide accurate information on long-term outcome.

A critical point is the potential utility of HVPG monitoring to guide therapy in this setting. HVPG can be used to treat non-responders with more intensive drug combinations to achieve response. The addition of ISMN to non-responders to beta-blockers (60–70% of cases) increases the rate of response up to 40–50%. A recent study suggests that shifting to prazosin instead of ISMN, as combined therapy with beta-blockers, may achieve response in more than 70% of non-responders. HVPG monitoring also provides guidance for rescue therapies to avoid rebleeding in non-responders. The efficacy of EVL in this setting has been contradictory. EVL was not useful in an uncontrolled study in which non-responders were switched from beta-blockers to EVL. Similarly, a recent RCT has shown that the addition of EVL in non-responders to beta-blockers plus ISMN did not reduce rebleeding risk [14]. Better results were obtained when partial responders to beta-blockers plus ISMN (with a decrease in HVPG ≥ 10% and < 20%) had EVL in addition to drug therapy, obtaining a low rebleeding rate (of only 20%). In this study, non-responders were treated with TIPS and no rebleeding was observed. Unfortunately, this study did not include a control group. All these data suggest that HVPG monitoring may guide therapy effectively. However, whether its use may improve the outcome of patients still should be demonstrated by adequate RCTs.

References

1. de Franchis R (2005) Evolving consensus in portal hypertension. Report of the Baveno IV consensus workshop on methodology of diagnosis and therapy in portal hypertension. *J Hepatol* **43**:167–76.
2. Laine L, Cook D (1995) Endoscopic ligation compared with sclerotherapy for treatment of esophageal variceal bleeding. A meta-analysis. *Ann Intern Med* **121**:280–7.
3. Hou MC, Chen WC, Lin HC, *et al.* (2001) A new "sandwich" method of combined endoscopic variceal ligation and sclerotherapy versus ligation alone in the treatment of esophageal variceal bleeding: a randomized trial. *Gastrointest Endosc,* **53**:572–8.
4. Nakamura S, Mitsunaga A, Murata Y, *et al.* (2001) Endoscopic induction of mucosal fibrosis by argon plasma coagulation (APC) for esophageal varices: A

prospective randomized trial of ligation plus APC vs. ligation alone. *Endoscopy* **33**:210–15.

5. Gonzalez R, Zamora J, Gomez-Camarero J, *et al.* (2008) Meta-analysis: Combination endoscopic and drug therapy to prevent variceal rebleeding in cirrhosis. *Ann Intern Med* **14**:109–22.

6. Lo GH, Lai KW, Cheng JS, *et al.* (2000) Endoscopic variceal ligation plus nadolol and sucralfate compared with ligation alone for the prevention of variceal rebleeding: a prospective, randomized trial. *Hepatology* **32**: 462–5.

7. de la Peña J, Brullet E, Sanchez-Hernández E, *et al.* (2005) Variceal ligation plus nadolol compared with ligation for prophylaxis of variceal rebleeding: a multicenter trial. *Hepatology* **41**:572–8.

8. Villanueva C, Miñana J, Ortiz J, *et al.* (2001) Endoscopic ligation compared with combined treatment with nadolol and isosorbide mononitrate to prevent recurrent variceal bleeding. *N Engl J Med* **345**:647–55.

9. Lo GH, Chen WC, Chen MH, *et al.* (2002) Banding ligation versus nadolol and isosorbide mononitrate for the prevention of esophageal variceal rebleeding. *Gastroenterology* **123**:728–34.

10. Patch D, Sabin CA, Goulis J, *et al.* (2002) A randomized, controlled trial of medical therapy versus endoscopic ligation for the prevention of variceal rebleeding in patients with cirrhosis. *Gastroenterology* **123**:1013–19.

11. Romero G, Kravetz D, Argonz J, *et al.* (2006) Comparative study between nadolol and 5-isosorbide mononitrate vs. endoscopic band ligation plus sclerotherapy in the prevention of variceal rebleeding in cirrhotic patients: a randomized controlled trial. *Aliment Pharmacol Ther* **24**:601–11.

12. Cheung J, Zeman M, van Zanten S, *et al.* (2009) Systematic review: secondary prevention with band ligation, pharmacotherapy or combination therapy after bleeding from oesophageal varices. *Aliment Pharmacol Ther* **30**:577–88.

13. García-Pagán JC, Villanueva C, Albillos A, *et al.* (2009) Nadolol plus isosorbide mononitrate alone or associated with band ligation in the prevention of recurrent bleeding: a multicentre randomized controlled trial. *Gut* **58**:1144–50.

14. Lo GH, Chen WC, Chan HH, *et al.* (2009) A randomized, controlled trial of banding ligation plus drug therapy versus drug therapy alone in the prevention of esophageal variceal rebleeding. *J Gastroenterol Hepatol* **24**:982–7.

15. Zheng M, Chen Y, Bai J, *et al.* (2008) Transjugular intrahepatic portosystemic shunt versus endoscopic therapy in the secondary prophylaxis of variceal rebleeding in cirrhotic patients: meta-analysis update. *J Clin Gastroenterol* **42**:507–16.

16. García-Pagán JC, Caca K, Bureau C, *et al.* (2010) Early use of TIPS in patients with cirrhosis and variceal bleeding. *N Engl J Med* **362**:2370–9.

17. Orloff MJ, Isenberg JI, Wheeler HO, *et al.* (2009) Randomized trial of emergency endoscopic sclerotherapy versus emergency portacaval shunt for acutely bleeding esophageal varices in cirrhosis. *J Am Coll Surg* **209**:25–40.

18. Khan SA, Smith T, Williamson PR, *et al.* (2009) Portosystemic shunts versus endoscopic therapy for variceal rebleeding in patients with cirrhosis. *The Cochrane Library Issue* **1**:1–61.

19. Henderson JM, Boyer TD, Kutner MH, *et al.* (2006) Distal splenorenal shunt versus transjugular intrahepatic portal systemic shunt for variceal bleeding: A randomized trial. *Gastroenterology* **130**:1643–51.

20. Orloff MJ, Orloff MS, Girard B, *et al.* (2002) Bleeding esophagogastric varices from extrahepatic portal hypertension: 40 years' experience with portal-systemic shunt. *J Am Coll Surg* **194**:717–28.
21. D'Amico G, García-Pagán JC, Luca A, *et al.* (2006) Hepatic vein pressure gradient reduction and prevention of variceal bleeding in cirrhosis: A systematic review. *Gastroenterology* **131**:1611–24.

Baveno V Consensus Statements
Prevention of Rebleeding

Didier Lebrec and Candid Villanueva (Chairpersons), Norman D Grace, Peter Hayes, Gin-Ho Lo, Frederic Nevens and Tilman Sauerbruch Arkhipov

Time to start secondary prophylaxis
- Secondary prophylaxis should start as soon as possible from day 6 of the index variceal episode. (5;D)
- The start time of secondary prophylaxis should be documented.

Patients with cirrhosis
- Combination of beta-blockers and band ligation is the preferred therapy as it results in lower rebleeding compared to either therapy alone. (1a;A)
- Haemodynamic response to drug therapy provides information about rebleeding risk and survival. (1a;A)
- The addition of ISMN to beta-blockers may improve the efficacy of treatment in haemodynamic non-responders. (5;D)

Patients with cirrhosis who are unable or unwilling to be treated with variceal band ligation (VBL)
- Beta-blockers with isosorbide mononitrate is the preferred option. (1a;A)

Patients with cirrhosis who have contraindications or intolerance to beta-blockers
- Band ligation is the preferred treatment. (5;D)

Patients who fail endoscopic and pharmacological treatment for the prevention of rebleeding
- TIPS with PTFE-covered stents is effective and is the preferred option. Surgical shunt in Child-Pugh A and B patients is an alternative if TIPS is unavailable. (2b;B)
- Transplantation provides good long-term outcomes in appropriate candidates and should be considered. (2b;B) TIPS may be used as a bridge to transplantation. (4;C)

Patients who have bled from isolated gastric varices type I (IGV1) or gastro-oesophageal varices type 2 (GOV2)
- N-butyl-cyanoacrylate (1b;A) or TIPS (2b;B) are recommended.

Portal Hypertension V, 5th edition. Edited by Roberto de Franchis.
© 2011 Blackwell Publishing Ltd.

Patients who have bled from gastro-oesophageal varices type 1 (GOV1)

- May be treated with N-butyl-cyanoacrylate, band ligation of oesophageal varices or beta-blockers. (2b;B)

Patients who have bled from portal hypertensive gastropathy

- Beta-blockers (1b;A) should be used for prevention of recurrent bleeding.

Patients in whom beta-blockers are contraindicated or fail and who cannot be managed by non-shunt therapy

- TIPS (4;C) or surgical shunts (4;C) should be considered.

Variceal Bleeding, Infections and the Hepatorenal Syndrome

Richard Moreau

Inserm U773, Centre de Recherche Biomédicale Bichat-Beaujon CRB3, Université Denis Diderot Paris 7, and Department of Hepatology, Hôpital Beaujon, Clichy, France

Introduction

Variceal haemorrhage and bacterial infections are common complications of cirrhosis that can trigger not only the hepatorenal syndrome (HRS) but also other causes of acute kidney injury (AKI) [1–4]. This chapter will successively comment on causes of AKI that develop in patients with variceal haemorrhage or bacterial infections; diagnosis of HRS; treatment and prevention of HRS.

Causes of AKI
Definitions

AKI is a syndrome which associates an acute decline in glomerular filtration rate (GFR), alteration of extracellular fluid volume, electrolyte and acid-base homeostasis, and retention of nitrogenous waste from protein catabolism [1]. In the clinics, renal failure is recognized by high serum creatinine levels. Causes of AKI are divided into prerenal, intrarenal, and postrenal factors (Figure 1) [1,3]. Prerenal factors range from obvious renal hypoperfusion in patients with hypotension to more subtle renal hypoperfusion, such as that seen in patients with cirrhosis and type 1 HRS. Postrenal acute kidney injury is caused by the blockage of urinary flow. Intrinsic (intrarenal) causes of AKI can be divided into diseases of the vasculature, tubulointerstitium, and glomerulus. In cirrhosis, the most common causes of AKI are "prerenal failure" and ischaemic acute tubular necrosis (ATN) [1]. In other words, renal hypoperfusion can explain most cases of cirrhosis-associated AKI [1].

Prerenal AKI in patients with acute variceal haemorrhage

In this setting, prerenal AKI may result from intravascular volume depletion with hypotension or true hypovolaemic shock (Figure 2) [1]. Some patients who do not have shock may develop type 1 HRS whose mechanisms are unclear [1]. Systemic inflammation resulting from ischaemia/reperfusion may play a role [1]. On the other hand, although patients with variceal haemorrhage receive antibiotic prophylaxis, some of them develop severe

Portal Hypertension V, 5th edition. Edited by Roberto de Franchis.
© 2011 Blackwell Publishing Ltd.

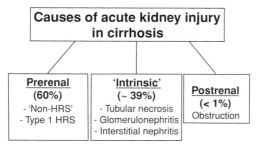

Figure 1 Causes of acute kidney injury in cirrhosis. HRS: hepatorenal syndrome.

bacterial sepsis causing AKI, including type 1 HRS (see below) [5]. Finally, one should have in mind that a significant proportion of patients with cirrhosis admitted for acute upper gastrointestinal haemorrhage have received non-steroidal anti-inflammatory drugs (NSAIDs) in the week preceding bleeding and NSAIDs may cause prerenal AKI (Figure 2) [1].

Prerenal AKI in patients with bacterial infection

In this setting also, there are different causes of AKI, including type 1 HRS (Figure 3). AKI occurs in patients with bacterial sepsis defined by proven or suspected bacterial infection plus the systemic inflammatory response syndrome (SIRS) [6]. Sepsis may trigger prerenal AKI via the following mechanisms: (a) intravascular volume depletion and hypotension as a result of fluid leakage caused by inflammatory injury of the microvasculature; (b) septic shock (in this case prerenal failure is very transient, see below); (c) intense renal vasoconstriction due to sepsis per se may precipitate type 1 HRS [1,6]. It should be noted that type 1 HRS may be precipitated not only by spontaneous bacterial peritonitis (SBP) but also by bacterial infections unrelated to SBP [7]. Finally, the intravascular administration of radio contrast agents to cirrhotic patients with bacterial sepsis may precipitate AKI [1].

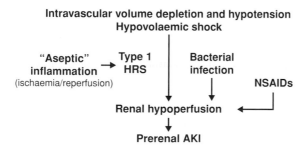

Figure 2 Causes of prerenal acute kidney injury in patients with cirrhosis and acute variceal haemorrhage. AKI: acute kidney injury; HRS: hepatorenal syndrome; NSAIDs: non-steroidal anti-inflammatory drugs.

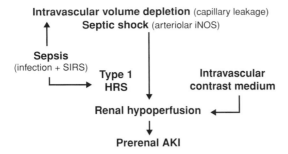

Figure 3 Causes of prerenal acute kidney injury in patients with cirrhosis and bacterial infections. AKI: acute kidney injury; HRS: hepatorenal syndrome.

Ischaemic ATN

Prerenal AKI is a pre-ischaemic state which is reversible if renal perfusion is restored by the appropriate treatment. However, prerenal AKI may progress very rapidly to ischaemic ATN in patients with hypovolaemic shock or septic shock [1,8]. In the absence of shock, the progression to ATN may be due to the absence of or delayed appropriate treatment [1]. Lesions of afferent arterioles, such as endarteritis or arteriolosclerosis are common in patients with cirrhosis without shock [9] and their presence correlates with that of acute tubular necrosis [9]. These findings are consistent with the fact that patients with lesions of afferent arterioles are prone to develop ischaemic ATN (the so-called "normotensive ischaemic ATN") for slight decreases in arterial pressure because of an impaired GFR [10].

Other "intrinsic" causes of AKI

They occur in patients with specific bacterial infections. For example, some cases of AKI due to post-infectious glomerulonephritis have been shown in cirrhotics with infection of the oropharynx or soft tissues [1]. AKI may also complicate acute pyelonephritis [11]. Together, these findings indicate that there are several possible causes of AKI in patients with cirrhosis and bacterial infection.

Diagnosis of HRS

It may be difficult to distinguish type 1 HRS from other causes of AKI [1].It has been suggested that urine indices (urine osmolality, urinary sodium concentration and fractional excretion of sodium) may help distinguish prerenal failure (including type 1 HRS) from tubular necrosis [1,8]. The tubular ability to reabsorb sodium and to concentrate urine is preserved in prerenal azotaemia and impaired in tubular necrosis [1,8]. Patients with prerenal failure have low urinary sodium concentrations (below 20 mmol/L) and elevated urine osmolality (higher than 500 mOsm/kg). Patients with tubular necrosis have high urinary sodium concentrations (above 40 mmol/L) and urine osmolality below 350 mOsm/kg. However, the urinary sodium concentration may be low early in the course of certain processes that lead to tubular necrosis such as sepsis, exposure to radio contrast agents or obstruction [1,8]. In addition, some cases of HRS with elevated urinary sodium concentrations have been reported [1]. Therefore, the International Ascites Club (IAC) has suggested using the following major diagnostic criteria to identify type 1 HRS [12,13]:

- Presence of decompensated cirrhosis
- A doubling of serum creatinine to a level > 2.5 mg/dL in less than two weeks
- No improvement of serum creatinine with diuretic withdrawal and volume expansion with intravenous albumin (20% solution)
- Absence of shock
- No current or recent nephrotoxic agent
- Absence of parenchymal kidney disease: proteinuria < 500 mg/day, red cells < 50 HPF, normal renal ultrasonography).

A recent study has analysed renal biopsy-specimens obtained by the transvenous route in cirrhotics who had high serum creatinine levels, proteinuria < 500 mg/day, no haematuria, and normal renal ultrasonography [9]. The results showed that these patients had unsuspected parenchymal lesions, among which glomerular and acute tubulointerstitial lesions [9]. These findings suggest three comments: first, IAC diagnostic criteria should be revised; second, renal biopsy may be useful for the diagnosis of AKI in patients with cirrhosis; and third, there is a need to develop biomarkers of renal lesions in patients with cirrhosis and AKI.

Treatment of type 1 HRS

This has been reviewed elsewhere [1,14]. Although the best treatment for HRS is liver transplantation, patients with HRS who are transplanted have more complications and a higher in-hospital mortality rate than those without HRS [1]. Therefore, in patients with HRS, it might be better to treat renal function abnormalities before liver transplantation [1]. It is important to note that HRS treatment should be started very early to avoid the progression of prerenal AKI to ischaemic ATN. It is an important point because to date there is no specific treatment for ATN [1]. In other words, one goal of early treatment of type 1 HRS is to prevent the development of ATN.

There is a strong rationale based on HRS pathophysiology (Figure 4), for using splanchnic vasoconstrictors in patients with type 1 HRS. Randomized clinical trials have shown that treatment with a combination of the vasopressin analogue terlipressin and intravenous albumin improved renal function in patients with type 1 HRS (Table 1) [15–19]. Predictors of terlipressin-induced improvement of renal function have been identified, including: lower MELD scores at the time of HRS diagnosis; significant pressor response to terlipressin; at least three days of terlipressin therapy; and lower creatinine levels at the time of HRS diagnosis [20,21]. This latter finding supports the early start of terlipressin therapy.

Other studies (with only two randomized trials, see Table 1) suggest that vasoconstrictor therapy with noradrenaline (combined with albumin) [18,19,22] or midodrine (combined with octreotide and albumin) [23–25],

Table 1 Characteristics of randomized studies using vasoconstrictor therapy in patients with hepatorenal syndrome*

Study Characteristics	First Author (reference) Solanki [15]	Sanyal [16]	Martin-Llahi [17]	Alessandria [18]	Sharma [19]
Patients with type 1 HRS, n	24	112	33	9	32
Patients with type 2 HRS, n	0	0	13	13	0
Study design	Single-blind, randomized, placebo-controlled – 12 patients assigned to terlipressin (1 mg/12 h IV) – 12 patients assigned to placebo	Double-blind, randomized, placebo-controlled – 56 patients assigned to terlipressin (1–2 mg/6 h IV) – 56 patients assigned to placebo	Open-label, randomized – 23 patients assigned to terlipressin (1–2 mg/4 h IV) plus albumin – 23 patients assigned to albumin alone†	Open-label, randomized – 12 patients assigned to terlipressin (1–2 mg/4 h IV) – 10 patients assigned to noradrenaline (0.1–0.7 μg/kg.min IV)‡	Open-label, randomized – 16 patients assigned to terlipressin (0.5–2 mg/4–6 h IV) – 16 patients assigned to noradrenaline (0.5–3.0 mg/h)
Concomitant IV albumin administration	All patients received albumin during follow-up (dose not specified)	All patients received albumin during follow-up (dose not specified)	All patients received albumin during follow-up (1 g/kg on day 1, then 20–40g/day)	All patients received albumin during follow-up – terlipressin group: 46 ± 10 g/day§ – noradrenaline group: 56 ± 4 g/day§	All patients received albumin during follow-up (20g daily)
Study endpoint Proportion of patients reaching the endpoint of HRS reversal (%)	HRS reversal – terlipressin: 42 – placebo: 0	HRS reversal – terlipressin: 34 – placebo: 13	HRS reversal – terlipressin: 35 – no treatment: 5	HRS reversal – terlipressin: 83 – noradrenaline: 70	HRS reversal – terlipressin: 50 – noradrenaline: 50
Proportion of patients with adverse events (%)	25 (terlipressin-related)	9 (terlipressin-related)	17 (terlipressin-related)	0 (in both groups)	– terlipressin: 6 – nordrenaline: 6

*HRS means hepatorenal syndrome; type 1 is the acute form of HRS and type 2 the "chronic" form of HRS, according to the definition provided by the International Ascites Club [12]. IV means intravenous. Plus-minus values are means ± SD. To convert values for creatinine to micromoles per litre, multiply by 88.4

†In the study by Martin-Llahi et al. 14 patients (60%) with type 1 HRS were randomly assigned to receive terlipressin plus albumin and 19 patients (83%) with type 1 HRS were randomly assigned to albumin alone [17]

‡In the study by Alessandria et al. 4 patients (42%) with type 1 HRS were randomly assigned to receive terlipressin and 4 patients (40%) with type 1 HRS were randomly assigned to receive noradrenaline [18]

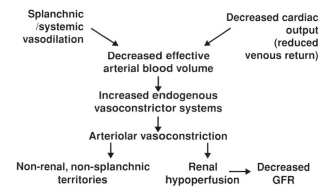

Figure 4 Pathophysiology of type 1 hepatorenal syndrome is the rationale for using splanchnic vasoconstrictors for the pharmacological treatment of this syndrome. GFR: glomerular filtration rate.

improves renal function in patients with HRS. On the other hand, therapies such as molecular adsorbent recirculating system (MARS) (eventually combined with intermittent venovenous haemofiltration) are under evaluation in patients with type 1 HRS [reviewed in Refs 1 and 14].

Prevention of type 1 HRS
Patients with acute variceal haemorrhage
Little is known on the impact of the standard care of haemorrhage on the development of type 1 HRS. Standard care associates antibiotic prophylaxis, optimization of extracellular fluid volume, administration of vasoactive drugs, endoscopic therapy and eventually TIPS. It should be noted that the use of standard care has been associated with an increase in in-hospital survival [26], suggesting that this beneficial effect may be at least in part related to a decrease in HRS occurrence.

Patients with bacterial infections
An open-label randomized clinical trial has shown that the administration of a combination of cefotaxime (a third-generation cephalosporin) plus intravenous albumin to patients with SBP significantly decreased the incidence of HRS and mortality [27]. The effect of intravenous albumin in patients with bacterial infection unrelated to SBP is still unknown. However, there are two randomized clinical trials that have addressed this question: one is completed and the other is still recruiting.

Primary prophylaxis of SBP
A randomized, double-blind, placebo-controlled trial of oral norfloxacin (400 mg/day) has been performed in patients with advanced cirrhosis, that is, low protein ascites (< 15 g/L) and liver failure or impaired renal function. In these patients, norfloxacin was found to significantly reduce at one year

the risk of SBP and HRS [28]. In addition, norfloxacin improved the three-month and one-year probability of survival compared to a placebo [28].

Pentoxifylline for patients with advanced cirrhosis

A large multicentre, randomized, double-blind, placebo-controlled trial of pentoxifylline (1,200 mg/day p. o.) has been conducted in patients with Child class C cirrhosis [29]. In these patients, pentoxifylline was found to significantly reduce the risk of development of HRS at six months. The mechanisms for this are unknown. Interestingly, in this trial, pentoxifylline was found to reduce the risk of bacterial infections at two months but not at six months, suggesting that the drug prevented the development of HRS independently of its effects on bacterial infections [29]. The effects of pentoxifylline in advanced cirrhosis may be related to its anti-inflammatory properties [29].

Conclusions

Patients with variceal haemorrhage and/or bacterial infections, are prone to develop AKI via different mechanisms, including HRS. The diagnosis of HRS is often difficult and new diagnostic tools should be developed. Specific treatment of HRS (i.e. terlipressin plus intravenous albumin) should be started very rapidly to avoid progression to acute tubular necrosis. Prevention of HRS can be achieved by different approaches.

References

1. Moreau R, Lebrec D (2003) Acute renal failure in patients with cirrhosis: perspectives in the age of MELD. *Hepatology* **37**:233–43.
2. Thabut D, Massard J, Gangloff A, *et al.* (2007) Model for end-stage liver disease score and systemic inflammatory response are major prognostic factors in patients with cirrhosis and acute functional renal failure. *Hepatology* **46**:1872–82.
3. Garcia-Tsao G, Parikh CR, Viola A (2008) Acute kidney injury in cirrhosis. *Hepatology* **48**:2064–77.
4. Ginès P, Schrier RW (2009) Renal failure in cirrhosis. *N Engl J Med* 361:1279–90.
5. Cárdenas A, Ginès P, Uriz J, *et al.* (2001) Renal failure after upper gastrointestinal bleeding in cirrhosis: incidence, clinical course, predictive factors, and short-term prognosis. *Hepatology* **34**:671–6.
6. Gustot T, Durand F, Lebrec D, *et al.* (2009) Severe sepsis in cirrhosis. *Hepatology* **5**:2022–33.
7. Terra C, Guevara M, Torre A, *et al.* (2005) Renal failure in patients with cirrhosis and sepsis unrelated to spontaneous bacterial peritonitis: value of MELD score. *Gastroenterology* **129**:1944–53.
8. Thadhani R, Pascual M, Bonventre JV (1996) Acute renal failure. *N Engl J Med* **334**:1448–60.
9. Trawalé JM, Paradis V, Rautou PE, *et al.* (2010) The spectrum of renal lesions in patients with cirrhosis: A clinicopathologic study. *Liver Int* **30**:725–32.
10. Abuelo JG (2007) Normotensive ischemic acute renal failure. *N Engl J Med* **357**:797–805.

11. Fasolato S, Angeli P, Dallagnese L, *et al.* (2007) Renal failure and bacterial infections in patients with cirrhosis: epidemiology and clinical features. *Hepatology* **45**:223–9.

12. Arroyo V, Ginès P, Gerbes AL, *et al.* (1996) Definition and diagnostic criteria of refractory ascites and hepatorenal syndrome in cirrhosis. *Hepatology* **23**:164–76.

13. Salerno F, Gerbes A, Ginès P, *et al.* (2007) Diagnosis, prevention and treatment of hepatorenal syndrome in cirrhosis. *Gut* **56**:1310–18.

14. Moreau R, Lebrec D (2006) The use of vasoconstrictors in patients with cirrhosis: type 1 HRS and beyond. *Hepatology* **43**:385–94.

15. Solanki P, Chawla A, Garg R, *et al.* (2003) Beneficial effects of terlipressin in hepatorenal syndrome: a prospective, randomized placebo-controlled clinical trial. *J Gastroenterol Hepatol* **18**:152–6.

16. Sanyal AJ, Boyer T, Garcia-Tsao G, *et al.* (2008) A randomized prospective double-blind placebo-controlled trial of terlipressin for type 1 hepatorenal syndrome. *Gastroenterology* **134**:1360–8.

17. Martín-Llahí M, Pépin MN, Guevara M, *et al.* (2008) Terlipressin and albumin versus albumin in patients with cirrhosis and hepatorenal syndrome. A randomized study. *Gastroenterology* **134**:1352–9.

18. Alessandria C, Ottobrelli A, Debernardi-Venon W, *et al.* (2007) Noradrenalin vs. terlipressin in patients with hepatorenal syndrome: a prospective, randomized, unblinded, pilot study. *J Hepatol* **47**:499–505.

19. Sharma P, Kumar A, Sharma BC, *et al.* (2008) Noradrenaline versus terlipressin in the treatment of type 1 hepatorenal syndrome: a randomized controlled trial. *Am J Gastroenterol* **103**:1689–97.

20. Colle I, Durand F, Pessione F, *et al.* (2002) Clinical course, predictive factors and prognosis in patients with cirrhosis and type 1 hepatorenal syndrome treated with terlipressin: a retrospective analysis. *J Gastroenterol Hepatol* **17**:882–8.

21. Nazar A, Pereira GH, Guevara M, et al. (2010) Predictors of response to therapy with terlipressin and albumin in patients with cirrhosis and type 1 hepatorenal syndrome. *Hepatology* **51**:219–26.

22. Duvoux C, Zanditenas D, Hezode C, *et al.* (2002) Effects of noradrenaline and albumin in patients with type 1 hepatorenal syndrome: a pilot study. *Hepatology* **36**:374–80.

23. Angeli P, Volpin R, Gerunda G, *et al.* (1999) Reversal of type 1 hepatorenal syndrome with the administration of midodrine and octreotide. *Hepatology* **29**:1690–7.

24. Wong F, Pantea L, Sniderman K (2004) Midodrine, octreotide, albumin, and TIPS in selected patients with cirrhosis and type 1 hepatorenal syndrome. *Hepatology* **40**:55–64.

25. Esrailian E, Pantangco ER, Kyulo NL, *et al.* (2007) Octreotide/midodrine therapy significantly improves renal function and 30-day survival in patients with type 1 hepatorenal syndrome. *Dig Dis Sci* **52**:742–58.

26. Carbonell N, Pauwels A, Serfaty L, *et al.* (2004) Improved survival after variceal bleeding in patients with cirrhosis over the past two decades. *Hepatology* **40**:652–9.

27. Sort P, Navasa M, Arroyo V, *et al.* (1999) Effect of intravenous albumin on renal impairment and mortality in patients with cirrhosis and spontaneous bacterial peritonitis. *N Engl J Med* **341**:403–9.

28. Fernández J, Navasa M, Planas R, *et al.* (2007) Primary prophylaxis of sponta-neous bacterial peritonitis delays hepatorenal syndrome and improves survival in cirrhosis. *Gastroenterology* **133**:818–24.

29. Lebrec D, Thabut D, Oberti F, *et al.* (2010) Pentoxifylline does not decrease short-term mortality but does reduce complications in patients with advanced cirrhosis. *Gastroenterology* **138**:1755–62.